Narcissism

and

Intimacy

A NORTON PROFESSIONAL BOOK

NARCISSISM
and
INTIMACY

LOVE AND MARRIAGE
IN AN AGE OF CONFUSION

MARION F. SOLOMON, Ph.D.

W. W. NORTON & CO, INC.   NEW YORK   LONDON

Published simultaneously in Canada by Penguin Books Canada Ltd.,
2801 John Street, Markham, Ontario L3R 1B4

Printed in the United States of America.

Library of Congress Cataloging-in-Publication Data

Solomon, Marion Fried.
   Narcissism and intimacy : love and marriage in an age of confusion
   / Marion F. Solomon. — 1st ed.
      p.   cm.
   ''A Norton professional book''—P.
   Bibliography: p.
   1. Narcissism. 2. Love—Psychological aspects. 3. Marriage-
-Psychological aspects. 4. Interpersonal relations. 5. Marital
psychotherapy. I. Title.
RC553.N36S65 1989
616.89'156—dc 19   88-21981
                                           CIP

ISBN 0-393-70057-7

W. W. Norton & Company, Inc., 500 Fifth Avenue, New York, N. Y. 10110
W. W. Norton & Company Ltd., 37 Great Russell Street, London WC1B 3NU

  2 3 4 5 6 7 8 9 0

To my husband, Matthew,
and my children, Bonnie and Glenn

Contents

Acknowledgments

Many friends and colleagues have read various sections of this book and have given me feedback about how the issues presented here could be recognized in the relationships they saw in treatment sessions and sometimes in their own lives. They have helped me to clarify my own thinking and to them I owe a great debt of gratitude.

To the patients who have given me permission to write about the hurts and fears that they have suffered, and who have willingly shared with me what has happened to them since treatment was terminated, I give my profound thanks. I have been most careful to assure that identifying information has been sufficiently altered so that their confidentiality is protected.

Special thanks to James Grotstein and Joan Lang, my co-editors on the two-volume *The Borderline Patient*. The hundreds of hours that were spent together attempting to answer the question "What is a borderline?" sparked my thinking about a subject basic to this book, "What is a narcissist?" I am indebted to them also for encouraging me to apply what we were learning to my writing about conjoint treatment of couples.

I wish to express my great appreciation to several experts in specialized subjects related to this book, who read and critiqued various chapters regarding which they have particular knowledge: Pearl Brown on countertransference and projective identification as tools of empathy; Ivan Gabor on the dynamics of couples as a group; Althea Horner on developmental issues in relationships; Robert Langs on conscious and unconscious communication; Arthur Malin on self psychology and affectivity; Joyce McDougall on defenses of mind and body.

Two therapists who are themselves experts in treating families and couples have helped me greatly by reading through versions of this manuscript to give me extremely valuable feedback: Rena Friedman, for her psychodynamically oriented approach, and Nancy Weiss for her family systems approach to treatment of marital problems. I thank also Anthony Caputo, who has kept me apprised of new medical research suggesting biological and genetic influences on development.

I have also been fortunate to have friends who expressed an interest in seeing this work in progress, who reviewed very early versions, and who related to me how the ideas affected their own thinking about relationships. For their time and generous responsiveness I thank Mary Von Asp, Caron Broidy, Nomi Morelli, and David Fried.

My thanks to Anthony Gerard who provided editorial commentary and early structuring of this manuscript. I am grateful also to Steve Levine, computer consultant extraordinaire, who on several occasions rushed over to save sections of this manuscript from being irretrievably lost deep in the belly of the computer.

I thank Ruth Mitchell, my guide and mentor in writing, for providing the principles by which to structure a book and by encouraging me to finally finish this book so that I might begin another.

These acknowledgments would not be complete without expressing my gratitude to my editor, Susan Barrows at W. W. Norton, who recognized the small seed of an idea in a short manuscript sent to her several years ago. It was her patience, direction, questions, and encouragement that turned some basic ideas into this book.

Throughout the process of thinking, discussing and writing I have been fortunate to have the interest and response of my daughter and professional colleague, Bonnie Solomon Mark, and son, Glenn Solomon. They have engaged in many dialogues with me over the years on the subject of love and marriage in contemporary culture, which have been a source of great pleasure as well as a learning experience.

More than anyone, my husband Matthew Solomon has been a mainstay, a source of constant encouragement and loving support. His influence is pervasive throughout the book.

Introduction

This book was originally conceived as a way of understanding the issues commonly seen in marital therapy. Those who read the manuscript as it was progressing pointed out that the descriptions of the underlying needs and conflicts of couples were applicable not only to marriage, but to all intimate relationships, unmarried and married, male and female, heterosexual and homosexual. We live in a world in which intimacy is hard to find and even harder to maintain. Not everyone is married, but everyone needs the sustenance of loving, intimate others.

When I entered the field of mental health in the sixties, I found myself in the midst of a revolution. Manners, values, and sexual morality seemed in constant flux. I watched friends and colleagues throw themselves into each new idea, therapeutic theory and growth potential, only to come away feeling angry, disappointed, and lonely. At the same time many who were experiencing marital or family problems were turning to psychotherapists in their search for fulfillment and meaning, the mental health profession was going through an identity crisis of its own.

For many, psychoanalysis was considered passé, the subject of jokes. The humanistic psychologists' call for greater acceptance of the self was fast providing the underpinnings for the narcissism of the "me generation." Pseudo-psychologies, cult-like in their recruitment of new prospects, offered a quick cure for those dissatisfied with their lives. Meanwhile, new therapies were on the rise.

It is now evident that the turmoil of the sixties and seventies fostered an atmosphere that has been very damaging to relationships. Some important things were missing from the new psychologies. Commitment lost its virtue, as marriage came to be viewed as confining and detrimental to personal growth. Many believed that the ties that bind must be loosened and, if they interfered with personal development, cut.

The divorces and unhappy relationships of friends and colleagues saddened me. I wanted to understand what was destroying the connections between husbands and wives, parents and children, friends and lovers, and to use my skills to help not only individuals but also relationships. Out of a basic knowledge of psychoanalysis and family systems theory, I came to a working understanding of how patterns of behavior and interpersonal experience are fixed as we are growing up and then replayed in adult relationships.

Since it seems easy to avoid dissatisfaction in marriage through divorce, people sometimes have little incentive to resolve their difficulties through understanding what has made love turn to boredom, indifference, or hate. Now we are being told that the failures of compatibility and commitment lie within certain men who have difficulty with relationships. Meanwhile, women continue to blame themselves for their failure to find or keep a loving man as an intimate partner in marriage. Therapists' offices are flooded with women trying to find out why they are distancing themselves from all the good, available men. The stress on personal growth at all costs associated with the "me" generation, the belief in the joy of free and equal lovemaking of the sexual revolution, and the "you can have it all" of the more intoxicating extremes of the feminist movement remain, even as we come to acknowledge a new awareness of the need for significant interpersonal connections.

This book is based upon the premise that good relationships are the backbone of emotional health. In our society, more than in the past, marriage is given the task of meeting essential human needs for emotional connection. Yet, because of a number of converging factors, including the messages that society sends us, the emotional failure between parents and children, and the history of failed relationships that today has become part of the life of many, a great number of individuals suffer from a narcissistic vulnerability that permeates all of their close relationships. Narcissistically vulnerable individuals desperately wish to be involved in a relationship but have expectations of giving and getting that almost invariably lead to disappointment for themselves and their partners.

Therapists and patients alike seem caught in the confusing demands, in the devaluation and even the denial of important realities; sometimes it appears that we have become the blind leading the blind. There is no evidence that the love relationships of therapists are any more stable or emotionally secure than those of any other professional group in our society. Therapists search for answers within themselves—they go into therapy, they read books, and they write books. But the revolving door of marriage, divorce, remarriage, divorce, alienation, and isolation that has permeated society has only recently begun to show signs of abating. Dangerous and deadly illnesses have forced many to assign new significance and value to intimacy. For the future well-being of our society, it would seem that there must be a reevaluation of the meaning of intimacy.

It is my deep conviction, after years of seeing couples in therapy, that the presenting issues revolving around money, work, or sex rarely cause the unhappiness between mates. Rather, misunderstandings, perceived as attacks, leave each partner feeling wounded, leading to a series of escalating retaliations and to defensive walls. Without understanding why, partners find that their loving feelings are deadened. Apathy or anger soon characterizes escalating exchanges in the relationship. When these patterns are carefully investigated in treatment, I have found that for one or both of the partners there has often been a history of early emotional failures and repeated injuries that left a residue of narcissistic vulnerability and defensive patterns.

Most people possess aspects of health as well as pathology. A variety of disturbances appear when an urgently felt need is not responded to, or when someone in a vulnerable state experiences a narcissistic wound. This can set in motion an escalation of defenses that interferes with functioning and manifests as increasingly pathological behavior. When there is a lack of affirmation or understanding, the relationship develops problems and the people involved begin to identify each other as narcissistic, emotionally lacking, or pathological.

When mates feel understood and confirmed by each other, they experience the relationship as a haven from the stressful world outside. The mental health field must include ways of helping to resolve issues that interfere with the maintenance of committed relationships. While therapists assist their patients in understanding and dealing with underlying needs and defenses, more than ever they need to support marriage partners' efforts to acknowledge and nurture one another in a benign environment.

This book has two parts. Part One examines the overall issues of narcissism in our society, in our families, and in our lives.

The beginning chapter identifies how in our present culture we are being indoctrinated in a narcissistically oriented view of relationships. Too often, modern expectations promise an idealized version of what love relations will provide. The cultural message is that we must be independent and autonomous individuals as a prerequisite for involvement in intimate relationships. By looking deeply within ourselves and discovering what we truly want, we are told, we can have all we desire. Expectations of entitlement pervade modern day marriages. All too frequently the result is disappointment and emotional distancing.

Family systems and marital relationships are the subject of Chapter 2. We see how the family, as the chief agent of socialization, provides the environment in which a personal model of interactions in relationships is established, and how these patterns are replayed throughout life.

The third chapter examines a range of narcissism in health and pathology, including the content of the primitive core within each of us. It introduces and describes a diagram that illustrates the internal events and experiences to which we regress in stressful situations. These internal experiences are on a continuum and are the precursors of narcissistic vulnerability. After a look at the transient narcissistic states that everyone experiences at times, I illustrate narcissistic manifestations by describing some situations drawn from my own work and from discussions with students and colleagues who shared their work in supervisory sessions. Various degrees of narcissistic vulnerability will be considered, from normal idealization and romantic love, at the higher level, to severe early narcissistic damage and its effect on relationships at the most archaic levels.

Chapter 4 traces the origins of narcissistic vulnerability through childhood development and considers how the developmental sequences in early life become building blocks of a lifetime of relationships. Chapter 5, the final chapter of Part One, considers affective response and defenses and includes a diagram outlining various levels of affects, emotions, and feelings that are experienced in times of narcissistic vulnerability and overwhelming injury.

Part Two focuses on understanding and repairing relationships that are damaged by issues of narcissistic vulnerability. It begins with descriptions of presenting problems, which are extremely varied. It also examines their underlying causes, which frequently seem to be variations on the basic theme of narcissistic injury. Two chapters, 6 and 7, describe marital problems and their behavioral manifestations. In Chapter 8 I discuss initial considerations in the treatment of couples, describe marital therapy as a model of treatment, and consider some issues that the therapist must ponder before deciding to work in a conjoint mode with couples. Chapter 9 describes marital therapy sessions as a "holding environment." Such a safe containing arena is needed to provide an island of safety while difficult internal and external issues emerge and are worked on in the relational space between husband and wife.

Chapter 10 is devoted to modes of interactional communication, verbal and nonverbal, which play such a large role both in marriage conflicts and in therapy. Finally, Chapter 11 discusses the therapist's own part in the situation through countertransference and empathy, as well as the role of the therapist as an advocate for the marriage.

In times when social pressures force a narcissistic world view on us, a marriage can be constructed as a safe place for two people to support each other. It can be a place where instead of pressure there is permission and acceptance. As such, it stands in opposition to our narcissistic culture, and thus requires a high degree of conscious understanding and clear communication. This book is intended to contribute to both.

Narcissism

and

Intimacy

PART ONE

CHAPTER 1

Love and Marriage in a Narcissistic Society

Many of the men and women I see in my psychotherapy practice are deeply disappointed in their relationships, their partners, and their lives. Expectation and reality do not match; instead they collide. Therapists' consulting rooms are filled with men and women who suffer because, in the confusing circumstances that prevail in our society, they cannot find a loving mate and a comfortable marriage. In my office I listen to men wondering why they cannot find the kind of woman they want to marry, and to women asking where all the good men have gone. "How do I get my man to make a commitment?" is a lament often voiced by women who hope that through therapy they will find the answers.

It is no wonder that there is an urgent search for answers. It seems increasingly difficult for people to enter and maintain loving relationships. The "culture of narcissism" (Lasch, 1979) has become a forerunner of an age of isolation, in which loneliness and emptiness seem pervasive for so many. There is a wish for simple answers to complex problems. Some therapists share with their patients a basic assumption prevalent in our society that men do not want to commit to marriage because of some basic defect such as a fear of commitment or an inability to experience emotions. Therapy based upon these beliefs tends to be repetitive, self-perpetuating, and not very helpful in the building of relationships.

The reality of marriage has probably never fit exactly with people's beliefs about it. These days, however, the disparity between reality and belief, custom and attitude, has become so great that it leads to much confusion. When the focus of life is on determining one's own needs and finding another who can fill those needs and wishes, any relationship is in danger of being flawed by narcissistic expectations. It is increasingly difficult for people to enter into loving relationships and to maintain them once they begin. Obligation to others as a primary value has become a concept either denied or distorted into a pseudo-love, a wish to embrace all mankind but no one in particular.

Many have come to expect fragile relationships that break easily, although they do not usually understand the nature of that self-fulfilling prophecy. Coupled with this belief is an increasing demand for effective independent functioning without emotional reliance on others. The result is an inability to invest freely in deep feelings for others.

Adults coming of age in the last quarter century have been socialized to have the kind of narcissistic world view that psychiatrists assert have replaced the classical neuroses as a leading cause of psychiatric disorder (Kohut, 1971). Pathology represents a heightened version of normality, according to Christopher Lasch (1979). Lasch quotes one of Otto Kernberg's patients: "The ideal relationship to me would be a two-month relationship. That way, there'd be no commitment."

THE EFFECT OF CHANGING PERCEPTIONS OF MARRIAGE ON MODERN RELATIONSHIPS

Many adults today who have gone through one or two marriages and one or two divorces—or who have witnessed the divorces of parents or friends—fear emotional investment in another person who could hurt them. There remains, though, an urgent search for someone to love—and for someone who will love back. In two such situations described below, the effect of cultural expectations and confusing messages about relationships made the search for love a precarious and ultimately unrewarding endeavor.

Debbie

When 43-year-old Debbie, a vivacious redhead with large green eyes, first walked into my office, she gave the impression that she "had it all together." However, as Debbie's story began to unfold, I realized that her controlled appearance was only a patina covering the angst that pervaded her life.

After four years of marriage, when Debbie was carrying their second child, her husband, Chuck, left her for the first time. His complaint was that he felt too constricted in the relationship. At that time the divorce laws in New York, where they lived, required there be just cause for divorce. Debbie refused to end the marriage. Ultimately, Chuck returned home and they resumed their relationship, but he was always restless.

Debbie devoted her life to her husband and children. She thought they were relatively happy. Later they moved to California and bought a house. Shortly after their eighteenth wedding anniversary, Chuck announced that he had fallen in love with another woman and wanted a divorce. Debbie again tried to hold the relationship together, but she no longer had any options. "No-fault" divorce laws permit one partner to decide unilaterally that there are irreconcilable differences and request dissolution of the marriage. The current divorce laws reflect cultural values. Personal happiness takes priority over previous commitment to another.

Debbie was granted half of the couple's assets and three years of spousal support, time to develop a skill to support herself and the three children. To split the assets, the house had to be sold. She had no steady income, no medical coverage, and no share in her husband's future social security benefits. As a result, the courts awarded the children to Chuck and his new wife, because the judge felt that they needed a solid home base. So, after 19 years of marriage, she found herself with no home, no children, and little income.

Immediately after the divorce, Debbie got a job and went out with many men who seemed to be quite interested in her. Although she invested her energies in one relationship after another, she always found herself wanting more commitment than the men in her life could or would give her. She went through a series of short-lived affairs, which left her with heartaches and herpes.

On dates she stopped talking about her work and started concentrating on the man's interests. She found herself purposely losing at tennis and recognized that in many ways she was subverting herself. The dishonesty started to exact its toll. She finally decided that she could not survive in relationships based on her willingness to take second place. Now, when Debbie meets a man, she keeps her distance because she doesn't want to get hurt. She expects very little and is seldom disappointed. While she waits for "that knight in shining armor," Debbie is throwing herself into a career so that she can take care of herself. She looks wonderful. She feels terrible.

Debbie is not unusual. She resembles many of the women seen in therapy. Some have been successful in their business careers and some have made careers as homemakers, but they are all confused and disappointed by their failure to have loving marriages.

Hal

Men have similarly frustrating experiences with relationships. Hal, who says that he hates being alone at night, has no idea how to meet the kind of woman he desires. He does not know Debbie, but he might once have been a perfect match for her. Tall and angular in appearance, intense in work and sports, 46-year-old Hal looks exactly like what he is, a scientist.

Hal does not see himself as the kind of man who would interest women. He is shy and somewhat absentminded—not at all a he-man. A child prodigy, he started college at 15 and never learned to make friends with people his own age. Although he has had two wives who fit his ideal, both marriages turned out to be calamities. He still does not feel comfortable dating, does not know what kind of woman he wants, and hates the shallowness of the women he meets in singles bars. While he is not unattractive, Hal believes that the kind of woman he dreams of does not want him. His wishes are high, his expectations at this point very low. He complains, "You have no idea the number of times I have gone to pick up a date that I had arranged several days before and found no one home . . . no call . . . nothing! Obviously, she found a better date."

Hal presently is thinking of marrying a woman he considers quite limited intellectually. His friends and family do not like her. Her tendency to horn in on his conversations with friends frustrates him, because he thinks that she contributes nothing. Nevertheless, the idea that she loves him and will do anything for him pleases him. He likes it when they are alone; he is able to read or work on his computer while she makes dinner, and their sex life is satisfying to him. He neither gives nor gets a great deal of pleasure in the relationship. Frustrated by what he characterizes as the "zoo" of the dating scene, Hal is ready to settle for a marriage that is reasonably comfortable and not too demanding.

Both Hal and Debbie would like to find a truly loving relationship, but both feel like giving up. The narcissistic culture in which they live encourages roles and expectations of oneself and of relationships that are conflicting, confusing, and often unrealistic. These expectations can be regarded as the myths of modern relationships, which will be discussed shortly.

CULTURAL HERITAGE AND THE INDIVIDUAL

Cultures develop particular styles of thought and modes of expression. How a person describes and explains what is being experienced is based upon the values, beliefs, and modes of thought peculiar to a society at a particular time and place (Harrison, 1985). Western civilization for the most part has tended toward self-celebration, a conception of man as the measure of reality and value. Oriental culture represents a harmony between man and nature—"alike, unreal and valueless in comparison to the realm of essence that exists independently of space and time" (Tomkins, 1987). "That other cultures have different ways of regarding time is not surprising. The Australian aborigines believed they could withdraw into a dream time where . . . ancestral figures coexisted with the present" (Harrison, 1985, p. 137). People reared in different cultures live in different sensory worlds—in other worlds of space and time.

In the societies of the past each differed from the others and each had lifestyles and modes of thought very different from our own, but in harmony with their own universe. Growing up in such a culture, people believed in their own internal experiences, just as we do in ours. We think of their mores, beliefs and values as mistaken based upon their lack of fuller knowledge. We tend to think of our own societal world views as more learned, mature, scientific. Among the great conceits of our modern age is the overriding belief that our culture, values and beliefs are the end result of a long line of progress.

THE EFFECT OF A CULTURE ON CHILDREARING PRACTICES

The culture as a whole influences how caretaking is provided, including expectations of the mothering role, views of the needs and responsibilities of children and adults, and the extent of development of the self. In addition, a culture's view of childrearing practices determines all other relationships within that society. Every society in history has had a unique view of how best to teach children—and in each this view has been seen as correct and better than those that came before. For centuries the emphasis on "breaking the will" of a child to cast out "original sin" (an emphasis that is the heritage of all in Western civilization) resulted in a method of childrearing that can only be viewed today as sadistic, abusive, and poisonous to innocent children.

Well into the twentieth century, the focus of child psychology was on methods of manipulating behavior rather than the basic need for consistent attachment and a loving relationship with "good enough" mothering (Winnicott, 1975). Not until John Bowlby's investigations, initiated in the 1940s, was the damage to current and later relationships of too early separation and loss explicitly reported (Bowlby, 1969).

Most people make the necessary inner adjustments to live within the boundaries of the values and beliefs of their culture. The internal world reflects the external universe. For example, when a young child cries, depending upon socialization and the family's position on expression of affect, the parents may pick the child up, converting the distress into a nurturing rewarding experience, ignore the crying, or insist that the crying stop immediately. The child, family, and society affect and are affected by each other in a process of dynamic equilibrium. The family is the chief agent of socialization into the economic-political-sociocultural system in which the child is born.

Where the society and family are benign, the inner and outer representational worlds generally fit well. This has often not been the case—witness, for example, murderous totalitarian regimes, the witchhunting society of 14th to 17th century Europe, or societies engaged in bitter civil or religious wars. Such societies do not allow for individuality or alternative individual world views. Even well-meaning and loving parents in such societies are forced to teach children distorted messages.

Sometimes events in a young child's life overshadow the ideo-affective position of the family and of society. A patient described his memories of being a young child of three, in Hungary during World War II, hiding in an attic for three years with his family before managing to escape to a safer place. Since crying, loud talking, or arguing with his brother or sister could endanger his family, all of his natural exuberance and aliveness had to be kept in check to protect others from the world outside. Blacks raised in the south 40 years ago had a similar experience. Failure to obey an order immediately could lead to a lynching. Parents taught their young children, particularly sons, to contain all feeling and emotion and never to talk back.

While there are large differences among classes in a population, no society permits total freedom of affect. In general the vocal or physical expression of rage, distress or terror must be contained. Males in our culture are particularly encouraged in the control of affect. Females, on the other hand, have permission to cry, but not to display angry or aggressive feelings. Societal values in this way have a major effect on psychological disturbances. Much of what is called "stress," Tomkins (1980) notes, is backed-up affect. It seems at the very least that substantial psychosomatic disease might be one of the prices of such systematic suppression and transformation of the innate affective responses (McDougall, 1986). Ambiguity about what affect "feels like" is another result, since much energy must be invested in defense against and transformation of affective response.

There is no question that different societies minimize or maximize aspects of family dynamics. There are societies that are socially structured so that it is assumed that all members are homogeneous. If this aspect of felt life is stressed, there is little need, and no societal pressure, to enhance the development of the self or of intersubjective relatedness. If, on the other hand, a society highly values the existence and the sharing of individual differences, then these aspects of development are facilitated by that society (Stern, 1985, p. 137). There are many cultures today (i.e., South American, Asian, and Middle Eastern) in which family relationships emphasize a closeness among relatives that would be considered by North American standards undue enmeshment and an impediment to personal growth.

THE DILEMMA OF MODERN RELATIONSHIPS

Rapid cultural changes in the decades following World War II produced confusion between responsibility to others and obligation to oneself. Personal obligations or feelings of responsibility toward parents, children, or marital partners seemed to have lessened. Young people began to see their parents' marriages and family interactions as the source of their own problems. As a result, many rejected conventional marriage and traditional concepts governing the reciprocity of love and esteem. Transient employment, regular changes of homes, the sexual revolution, and easier divorce laws made parent-child and husband-wife relationships a low priority. Commitment came to be viewed as a trap to keep an individual from fulfilling important self-determined goals.

We have been raised to expect that our lives can be busy, exciting, fulfilling, and materially successful. We believe that marriage should be part of that. Males and females alike seek loving, emotionally stable partners. In the idealized image of the modern American couple, the dual career team, the man takes more responsibility for the care of the children and the home than men have in the past and the woman takes more responsibility for financial support of the family than women have in the past. It is assumed that members of both sexes can "have it all"—a successful career and a happy family life. In the fantasy, everyone gets what he or she wants. But that is not what most men and women experience. Both men and women have lost the clear knowledge of what is expected of them, individually and in relationships. We are bombarded with a series of cultural myths that tell us that we can have it all, that we must be responsible to ourselves first, that a successful life depends more on financial success than on ethical or moral values. The myths of relationships permeate our lives with narcissistic expectations. In the following section, I describe eight of these modern myths.

MODERN MYTHS

1. The focus on the self as the most important component of one's existence leads to narcissism as a goal—not a pathology. The current "culture of narcissism" has as a basic aspect the *myth of entitlement*.

2. In general, we strive for independence and equate dependence with weakness and immaturity. This is supported by the *myth of autonomy*.

3. Many of us believe that if we find our "one true love," we will live "happily ever after." This is the *myth of romantic love*.

4. There is a misconception that women have a greater need to be in an intimate relationship than do men, and that women are healthier and happier when they are married, while men are better off when they are single. This is the *myth that the benefits of marriage are greater for women than for men*.

5. There is a common belief that the marriage rate is falling precipitously and that marriage may no longer be a viable institution. This is the *myth of marriage in decline*.

6. The sources of a large number of relationship problems have been based on misconceptions about what is normal and appropriate male and female behavior. These are *gender myths* that must be examined more closely.

7. There is a belief held by many today that women have a choice to work or stay home and that they are choosing to work for personal fulfillment. This is the *myth that women's liberation is the cause of social decline*.

8. Finally there is the belief that problems of marriage can be resolved by making divorce a less guilt-producing, fault-finding process. This is the *myth of positive divorce*.

The Myth of Entitlement

The self-centered narcissism of the "me generation" has not resolved the conflict between old attitudes and fantasies about marriage and newer ideas about men, women, and relationships. Nothing has replaced the values that came in the wake of sweeping social change. Although many people seek balance in their attitudes toward love and sex, they have not yet found ways to change the well-entrenched internal program that endorses narcissistic self-involvement as a means to fulfillment. As a result, they have trouble finding meaning in a maze of conflicting values, including demands that all unfairness and injustice be corrected immediately and that people be granted their rights to unconditional acceptance, nonjudgmental attitudes, and empathic understanding from both family and friends. While these are laudable goals, outside of the therapeutic consulting room they can become narcissistic entitlement demands.

Where appropriate roles in relationships are not clear, confusion increases and the ability to turn for support and comfort to others decreases.

Modern mythology produces the answers and the cultural leaders to provide temporary feelings of security. Rock stars, sports stars, super-heroes and anti-heroes provide pseudo-solutions to make the world seem a safer, more manageable place. Cultural messages all around us confirm a self-centered approach to living. Notoriety of any sort receives our rapt attention. People with narcissistic personalities are elevated to positions of eminence and power. Celebrities set the tone for appropriate behavior. Fame is valued above all else. We demand of our idealized media stars that they act in ways that reinforce a fantasy of narcissistic success, reflecting our collective wish to be vastly admired uncritically and without reservation, not for our accomplishments but simply for ourselves.

What seems to be distinctive about our times is that society sees narcissistic traits as a means to achieve an end, not as a problem. The result is that many people who have no diagnosed psychiatric disorder and who are relating with culturally reinforced ways of behaving seem to have feelings that are similar to those with narcissistic pathology. They feel cut off, empty, drained and unable to develop satisfying relationships with others, while desperately wishing to have someone with whom they can be close.

There has been but a whisper of a challenge to the current assumptions that we must take care of ourselves first, that only then can we fully be in a relationship with others. To do what one's partner wants instead of what is important to oneself usually appears to be a dangerous sacrifice of the self for a relationship.

> I do my thing, you do your thing
> I am not in this world to meet your needs;
> you are not in this world to meet my needs;
> If by chance we meet, it's beautiful
> If not, it can't be helped. (Perls, 1969)

Fritz Perls' motto, adopted enthusiastically by the "me generation," is a recipe for narcissism, with its concomitant loneliness and emptiness. For many people there is no longer a feeling that "we are in this together, for better or for worse." Instead, there is constant reevaluation of themselves, their mates, their relationships. Life becomes an exhausting round of questions, "Is this relationship giving me all that I want, need, and deserve? Might I get what I need by getting out and trying to find someone else who will give me more?" All too often, the decision has been on the side of giving up the relationship and seeking a more "perfect" love.

When partners are confused about what they may expect of each other emotionally, they often attribute the problem to some pathology of the other. Often the problem has been magnified by the methods that have evolved to deal with the inner emptiness experienced by so many. People have come to believe that they are entitled; they have a right to live life and have relationships totally on their own terms. But no relationship is free. On the contrary, constraints and responsibilities are integral to human interaction.

Many self-help programs, including those that purport to be therapeutic or are pseudo-religious, promote narcissistic entitlement demands. "You can have it all," they encourage. "Only the lack of clear conceptualizations of what you want keeps you from having it all." "Learn to communicate," "learn to chant," "become more assertive"—and all things will come to you. It is assumed that the only thing that keeps us from being or having exactly what we want is our own fear of going after it. While assertiveness can be a very helpful tool for self-development, assertive entitlement is a reversion to a primitive fantasy that "I am the center of the world," a fantasy acted upon by many today. That is why many people today exhibit symptoms of narcissistic pathology, particularly the sense of being automatically entitled.

The Myth of Autonomy

The result of pervasive narcissism is a new myth—that each person must be a whole unto him- or herself, autonomous and fulfilled without needing anything from others, before being able to be in a relationship. A healthy person, though, cannot be totally separate from others. Autonomy is a relative state requiring another person with whom we establish boundaries. Without others, there is no autonomy, only isolation.

Despite attempts in the past few years to glorify the individual and downplay the importance of relationships, there is ample evidence that people need people to survive, not just to provide services, but to offer love and a sense of being valued. The importance of love for our well-being is well documented. Infants die if they are not physically held; so may adults. "The most dangerous thing in the world is not to be weak—we all manage to survive the ludicrous weakness and inadequacy of our infancy: the most dangerous thing in the world is to be unloved" (Gaylin, 1984, p. 29).

A major problem today was identified by Andreas-Salome (1962), when she pointed out the contradictory tendencies of narcissists to search for individuality at all costs and yet be unable to live outside of a continuing state of fusion. That apparent contradiction is the basis for a myriad of relationship problems. Yet, it is not a love of oneself that causes problems in relationships, but the remnant of narcissism inappropriately responded to, which leads to development of unrealistic defenses to protect vulnerable, frightened selves. Too often this is reinforced by a cultural milieu that encourages expendable relationships in service of material success. The result is a two-pronged assault on a basic human need to love and be loved.

The normal need for autonomy and differentiation described in considerable depth in the family therapy literature (see Chapter 2) has, for some time been distorted into an attitude of *self above all*. The psychotherapeutic accent on separation and differentiation results sometimes in increasing autonomy at the cost of mutuality and affectional bonds. "I don't want you to see a therapist," a new patient reported her husband as saying. "Someday you will come home and tell me that you are cured, you need your independence, and you want a divorce." His fears are not totally unreasonable in light of the prevailing societal mood for the past three decades.

The early experience of merger does not necessarily result in a loss of boundaries in later life. In fact, temporary states of merger are experienced by some couples as a most pleasurable aspect of a relationship. It is one aspect of a fulfilling sexual relationship with a loved other. More than that, it is a part of what makes up the relationship of "the heavenly twins" (Jackson and Lederer, 1968); that is, it fosters a feeling that each partner holds a part of the other.

The Myth of Romantic Love

In the past, marriage was an economic and social arrangement designed to give families the best chance of surviving and producing offspring. Children were needed to work farms, produce goods, and help with household tasks. Although power was unevenly divided, the customary division of labor gave both husband and wife roles in contributing to the welfare of the family. Marriage choices were made on the basis of what the partner could bring into the union. Companionship, happiness, and contentment, of course, were not uncommon in such marriages, but they were not the overriding consideration.

Over the last century, values in marriage have undergone a radical change. Marriage today is portrayed as being held together by the strength and significance of the couple's interpersonal relationship—a relationship based on mutual respect, affection, empathic understanding and friendship. Love and companionship are the basis for modern marriages; thus, the emphasis has drifted away from survival and economic security, which were a crucial element of marriage in earlier times.

The partnership concept has taken on new dimensions because of a continuing change in roles and expectations, and the emergence of new ways of viewing male-female relationships. The model of marriage in the late 1980s has shifted from a picture of two closely intertwined persons with clearly defined gender roles, who are part of an extended family, to a picture of two independent people with individual goals, styles and personalities.

In the same way that fulfillment of emotional needs has become the main purpose of family relationships, finding a perfect, permanent love has become the all-important quest of the single adult. If the first attempt at lasting love is not successful, one has the right, and even the obligation, to leave the relationship in order to find one's "true love."

Romantic love has become both the basis for mate selection and a potentially fatal trap of unattainable expectations. Disappointment often leads to an inability to give emotionally to the mate or the children, setting the stage for the cycle of emotional failure. Even for the child who has received a great deal of healthy emotional support from parents, the demands made of relationships easily lead to great disappointment when "true love" does not fulfill its promise.

The Myth that Marriage Benefits Women More than Men

The belief that women need and desire close relationships more than men do seems to me to receive little justification from the facts. Jessie Bernard (1972) has pointed out research evidence that counters the common notion that marriage is a less natural state for men than for women and that males contribute more and get less out of marriage than females.

While men have been railing against marriage for centuries, have cursed it and denegrated it, Bernard notes they never cease to want it and profit from it. Men choose to be married because "on almost every index— demographic, psychological or social," married men do better than their unmarried counterparts, suffer from fewer mental health impairments, have a lower suicide rate and a lower death rate from illness (p. 17).

The benefits of marriage to men, in fact, outweigh those to married women. Women who are married are more likely to seek treatment for physical and mental disorders than their unmarried sisters (Bernard, 1972). Bernard notes that more wives than husbands report marital frustration and dissatisfaction; more report negative feelings, consider their marriages unhappy, and have considered separation or divorce. The marriage relationship clearly fulfills important conscious and unconscious needs, since, despite unmet expectations and myriad disappointments, men and women continue to marry.

The Myth of Marriage in Decline

Sometimes it seems as though people change husband and wives as often as they change automobiles. The repeated rotation of partners leaves the impression that no one stays married any longer. It must be remembered, however, that 95% of American people marry (*New York Times*, October 24, 1983) and that over half of the marriages in this country are between people who have had only one partner. Of those who divorce 83% of the men and 75% of the women remarry (*New York Times*, October 24, 1985). Because of higher expectations about married life and the greater possibility that dissatisfaction will lead to divorce, those who remain wed are more likely to do so out of choice. Recently, there have been suggestions that women forgo marriage as it demands too much and offers too little (Hite, 1987). Yet the outpouring of current books on the subjects of love and marriage provides evidence of the continued desire for marriage on the part of adults today.

Despite the pain experienced by most people who divorce, marriage continues to be the relationship of choice for a majority of men and women today. This is because in our society a marital relationship is one of the few places that provides opportunities to meet important needs for intimacy and security. Until some alternative workable model emerges, the structure of marriage and family systems may change, but the institution of marriage itself is viable.

Gender Myths

Most psychiatric literature is written as though there were no such thing as gender differences (Lang, 1985). We still do not have good answers to questions about what is inherently male and what is inherently female. Are men innately action oriented and women emotionally oriented? Are differences based on our giving little boys toy guns and little girls dolls? Or do children demand certain objects because of certain innate characteristics or immutable psychological interactions?

Although males and females face the same basic existential problems in life, such as death, aloneness, insufficiency, imperfection, they deal with these problems in different ways. They experience and use love differently. For the female the passionate quest in life is interpersonal, romantic, and permanent. For the male it is heroic, the pursuit and achievement of power (Person, 1988).

In her book, *In A Different Voice* (1982), Carol Gilligan suggests that males and females face different developmental challenges. Even as she establishes her own identity as a woman, a girl maintains the close ties with her mother that were established in infancy. The female child identifies with the nurturing other and eventually learns that she too will grow up to have and care for babies. Her role in life is to repeat her earliest intimate experience as nurturer. As she comes to recognize her father, there is an awareness of otherness. Her relationship with her father is likely to be repeated for better or worse in the intimacy of a future marriage.

The male child has a different experience. At first he may identify with his mother. As awareness of others in his world expands, he becomes aware of his father. In normal development, the male child recognizes that he will not grow up to be a mother. In fact, to begin the process of identification with the father, he must separate himself from the mother. Although like father, the young boy recognizes that he is much smaller and cannot compete. The next hope is to become more like father by entering competition as he grows and becomes stronger.

To grow up male in our society is to engage in ongoing competition and to be measured constantly. How fast and far he can run, hit, throw a baseball, kick a football, how well he handles fights, the size of his penis — all identify the male self. Despite adult words about "how you play the game," for most males, as for their peers and their fathers, winning the game is the important thing, and defining the rules is the first part of winning. All games of schoolboys begin with selecting "captains" and being chosen last for the team is often recalled as the most humiliating experience of childhood.

There is also a basic difference in how children engage in games. When Gilligan (1982) studied the ways children played games, she found that girls had less need than boys to agree on specific rules. Boys are extremely rule-conscious, while girls are relatively tolerant of innovations in a game. Boys will spend a great deal of time arguing about the rules; girls will change to a new game instead. From fairly early on, females are reinforced for being connected and nurturing, while males are reinforced for engaging in thought and action.

Some men have been convinced that their "nonfeeling" reaction is a sign of a psychological problem, and have entered therapy to try to cure it. And, in fact, as close relationships are defined by such interchanges as verbal self-disclosure, expression of emotional reactions, a willingness to admit to loving feelings, most men do appear to have shortcomings (Levinson, 1978). However, the reality is that men do not lack feelings or deep unconscious affects and emotions, although many men do consider displaying feelings to be a weakness. They may be more comfortable dealing with feelings through action rather than emotional expression. As a way of demonstrating caring in a relationship a man may take a mentor role. Involvement and concern among men are demonstrated by a distinctive style of love that focuses on giving real and practical help, while a woman desires a display of emotion.

As I listen to discussions about relationship issues in group therapy (without spouses present), it is clear that men and women often operate in very different ways. Women enjoy intimate conversations with friends about every aspect of their lives, including problems in their relationships with their lovers and husbands. To men, discovering that their personal lives and habits are being discussed with others outside of the relationship is a source of great consternation. Men are much more cautious than women about sharing their inner thoughts and emotions—a source of many complaints by women, who see this as a sign of "not being in touch with feelings." Modern assessments of intimacy seem to be based upon a model of verbal sharing favored by women.

When men do communicate in a relationship they generally talk about their victories, achievements, success and power in competition with other men (Cancian, 1987). They share personal troubles and vulnerabilities only with an intimate partner. Men do confide in a mate when they feel assurance that it is absolutely safe to do so. I have heard a number of men say that they wish that they could discuss their fears and anxieties but usually find that sharing their burdens only makes their partner anxious. They worry about looking weak and keep their own counsel. Rarely do men talk about their marital or financial troubles with other men. Rather than talking about such things to a friend, they prefer a comfortable camaraderie, observing or participating together in activities or competitive sports events.

As I listen to men and women explain their views, I can understand how the differences often result in major problems in relationships. Therapists must work harder to ferret out the emotional responses of men, to hear what is not spelled out clearly or is discussed in derivative form. But they must also be careful not to assume that being in touch with emotions is a sign of psychological health. As noted in Chapter 3, feelings, emotions and affects are a complicated subject, and differences should not be seen as defects. The treatment chapters in the latter half of this book describe ways of translating the deeper levels of affect that are hidden in communications patterns.

Large groups in our society are being taught to suppress many of their basic feelings. For years it was educated women who had to submerge their own strength and power in submission to men. When women rebelled against this yoke of oppression and demanded equality, it sometimes resulted in the expectation of a role reversal. Men heard that they should get as much joy and pleasure out of nurturing children as women did. Caretaking of babies is a gender neutral experience, they were told. Men were expected to allow women into the domain of the competitive work world with positive regard and support. But often neither men nor women were comfortable with their newly assigned feelings.

Many men profess to desire equality in relationships between the sexes. Educated males in our society have acknowledged and accepted the fairness of these new rules, at least on the surface. To challenge them makes one a "male chauvinist pig" or a "redneck"—or whatever pejorative one might apply to someone who goes against the cultural norm. To accept, however, sometimes makes men appear weak to themselves, as well as to the women in their lives. They fear being labeled as inadequate and rejected. Other men who do not wish to give up the privileges enjoyed by the male sex may give only lip service to women's legitimate expectations. Their repressed feelings come out in a variety of ways, not the least of which is silent resistance to the relationships that women want.

As women have attempted to break old stereotypes that say women are weak, illogical and overly emotional, they maintain old stereotypes about men. Men are supposed to be strong, rational, sexually assertive, and fearful of commitment. Men work hard to protect this image because throughout their lives, from childhood through adult relationship, they get the message that they must be strong. Despite many changes in society, boys who do not demonstrate strength are called "sissies." Men who are gentle, sensitive, and easily able to show emotions are often labeled "wimps." "Don't be vulnerable. Don't be helpless or passive or sensitive," men have learned.

Many men today are confused about whether they want a wife to take care of them and their home or an economic helpmate. Being men, they do not talk much about their confusion. To many women who wonder what men want, the answer seems to be that men are unreasonable: They want nurturing and caretaking but they do not want commitment. They want women to be strong and able to take care of themselves and at the same time they want submissive, accommodating women who will listen to their problems and be supportive.

Successful adaptation to modern marriage seems to require, as Dicks suggested 20 years ago, "a blend of autonomy of the individual, an established sense of personal identity and ego strength, and a preservation of the capacity for dependence" (1967).

The Myth That Women's Liberation Is the Cause of Social Decline

The women's liberation movement began with a group of educated middle-class women who sought more intellectual and social stimulation than was available in the suburbs of post-World-War-II America. And they found a cause—the disparity between men and women's job opportunities and income, as well as overt and covert sexism.

While this battle was being fought, changing economic conditions were encroaching on decisions about employment for women. A job, which had always been a necessity for the working poor, increasingly was becoming a requirement for all but the very rich. Most men have never had a choice to work or to stay home. Most women no longer have a choice today.

According to the *Wall Street Journal*, 65% of mothers of school-aged children are employed (January 19, 1985). When there is a divorce, women's income and standard of living drops 73% while men's income and standard of living increase by 47% (Wallerstein, 1985). Women must be prepared to support themselves and often their children as well. To maintain a lifestyle comparable to that of their parents, most young marrieds must pool two incomes. Buying a home often means postponing children because both partners must work. Adequate childcare while parents are working is virtually unavailable for all but the most affluent young couples.

Many women recognize that achieving success in the business world may require their full energy and leave little or no time for relationships outside of their professional lives. A study of successful business people by the University of Michigan's School of Business Administration adds another perspective (Hildebrandt, 1986–1987, 1987). Men, indeed, seem to be able to have both career and family. The majority of men who become top business executives are married, but the majority of women who make it to the top are unmarried. Women have become increasingly aware of having to make a choice between running a business and running a family and home. Seldom do they have the option of marrying a helpmate who will assist in maintaining a satisfying home and family life.

Male executives have a distinct advantage over their female counterparts. The men in the Michigan study cited "maintaining a satisfying and well-run home" as the most important function of their partners. In addition, they indicated that they expected their wives to "offer emotional support," to "participate in company activities," and to "act as hostesses." There is no equivalent person to serve these functions for women, which is why I have heard many women executives say, "I need a wife."

When working women get home, they are tired and want to relax in a home that is a haven from the pressures of work; they want someone to soothe them and listen to their tales of the trials and successes of their day. Instead they face dinner to be made, laundry to be done, children's needs to be attended to, and a husband burdened by his own work pressures. Tired husbands and tired wives, with little reserve energy for the ordinary crises of everyday life, often find themselves saying, "What about me?"

Because of their new economic and social situation, women have less time, energy, or inclination to provide emotional support to the men in their lives. As they talk among themselves, women question why they should, since they may be carrying burdens at least as heavy as the ones carried by men, and perhaps heavier. While the goals of women's liberation are admirable, economic and social events have caused not a resolution, but added burdens.

The Myth of Positive Divorce

Some have proposed that the marriage contract be nonpermanent and subject to renewal at various points in the marriage. If partners grew and changed, then the relationship could be ended and new partners found. Assuming that marriage should last only as long as both partners find the relationship meaningful means that divorce should be pain-free and guilt-free. However, "no-fault" divorce, initiated by either partner at any point in the relationship, may leave the other, after many years of marriage, forced to live alone and begin life again.

Women, who more commonly come out on the short end of the divorce stick, have found themselves with no training, no employment history, no social security or insurance benefits. Abby, an angry and depressed member of a post-divorce therapy group, described her experience of uncomplainingly sharing the lean years and being left when it came time to share the "fat" years. She had put her husband through medical school by working as a secretary. When he graduated from school, he graduated from the marriage as well. He moved in with his office manager and they are now going to have a baby. "It's not fair," she said in despair, helpless to do anything about the fact that she earns less than one-third of his salary, while the court granted her one-half of their accumulated property, her car, and their bedroom set.

Joel and Lillian were married 14 years when he asked for a divorce to marry another. She discovered too late that all of his investments, including their home, were built upon a base of a moderate inheritance he had received from his father. All of the income that was earned during their marriage was used for living expenses. There was no community property, despite large real estate holdings accumulated over the years of their marriage. Although she was enraged, she could do nothing. She was told to consider herself fortunate that the court granted her three years of spousal support and tuition for school.

There has been a belief that children are better off in a divorced home than in a house dominated by unhappily wed parents. This may be true for some, when the home is filled with physical or emotional abuse. However, there is an emerging consensus that divorce constitutes a major disequilibrium in the lives of most children. A national survey of children reported that more than twice the number of children from divorced families than from intact families had seen a mental health professional (Zill, 1983). In another study it was reported that men and women whose parents divorced when they were young children or adolescents reported significantly more problems related to work, higher divorce rates, and higher levels of emotional distress than did their counterparts who grew up in intact families (Hetherington and Parke, 1979). Other research has indicated that children are at risk for developing social, emotional and behavioral problems that may first appear years after the divorce (Guidubaldi and Perry, 1985). The problems of children coming away from divorce include sadness, depression and poor self-esteem, as well as aggressive and antisocial problems (McDermott, 1970; Hetherington, Cox, and Cox, 1985).

The reality is that for those who decide to divorce, ending a relationship that began in loving hopefulness is extraordinarily painful; the grief resembles the response to the death of a loved one. "It was like having my skin torn off," said one person in group therapy, and everyone in the group recognized the feeling.

PROBLEMS IN THE SEARCH FOR INTIMACY

The search for intimacy inevitably implies the setting up of a system of mutually acceptable solutions to the problems of being together. Each partner comes from a different family regulated by a different storehouse of solutions to the stresses and common problems of living. Each has been indoctrinated with the values and beliefs of a particular historical place and time. Expectations and preexisting solutions inevitably enter into the building of the new system, conditioning it in various ways.

Each partner brings into the marriage a personal world view of how things ought to be as well as a developmental history that programs interpersonal roles of husband, wife, parent, children, friends, and community interaction. These are not experienced as personal values, beliefs and ways of seeing the world, but as truth and reality.

Currently we are going through a major transition in our thinking about relationships. Just as we have begun to believe that mature individuals might be capable of functioning in an independent manner without needing others to fulfill childlike dependency needs, we have come to recognize how lonely it can be. Coinciding with a new guardedness in sexual experimentation, there is a major shift back to commitment and monogamy in relationships.

The role of the therapist is to understand the internal world of both spouses as they present in words the closest approximation of their version and views, to recognize from verbal and nonverbal indications how they try to meld together these views, and to recognize how they attempt to resolve problems that occur when personal world views clash or when inner needs of either partner demand more than the other is able or willing to meet.

CHAPTER 2

Marriage as a System

Getting married requires the setting up of a system of mutually acceptable solutions to the problems of living together. Each partner comes from a different family regulated by a different storehouse of solutions to the stresses and common problems of living. These preexisting solutions inevitably enter into the building of the new system, conditioning it in various ways. In this chapter, we will look at the unique system set up by each marriage, how it works to support or tear down the individuals involved, and how damage occurs, as illustrated in some cases. We will also see what goes into some successful mutual accommodations.

Marriage embraces two individual subsystems that combine to form a new family system. The task of the spouses is to devise, consciously and unconsciously, a mutual working system that allows them to function comfortably without completely sacrificing the values and ideals they brought into the marriage. A new social order with its own structure and language develops through a process of trial and error. Partners influence each other and members of their respective birth families and are in turn influenced by their relatives-in-law.

Distortions of present reality based on early developmental experiences and the struggle for personal affirmation and confirmation are so interwoven into the process of establishing an identity as a couple that they are only dimly visible. The fate of the relationship depends on what happens when "the honeymoon is over" and in particular how the partners deal with the realization that many of their fantasy-based expectations are unlikely to come true. Marriage can foster growth and the establishment of a new level of individual functioning, or it can become a repository for old conflicts and unmet needs.

Bowen (1966) noted that, despite apparent differences in overt social functioning, people tend to marry those who are at the same basic level of personality differentiation, but who have opposite patterns of defensive organization. When such an experience is reenacted, a person who experienced early rejection or abandonment may choose a mate whose enmeshed family was engulfing. The former desires greater closeness in a relationship, while the latter struggles for more separateness. At the same time each reenacts what is known. Old patterns are repeated because the known, however unsatisfying, is more comfortable than the unknown, and is therefore less dangerous. Kubie (1956) notes that marital partners are selected in the hope that they will wipe out old pains or pay off old scores. Napier (1978), perhaps on a more pessimistic note, hypothesized that people tend to marry their worst nightmares.

Often one partner desperately wishes that the other would be responsive but gives no sign of such neediness, for fear of shameful exposure. Many never learned the basic skill of communicating needs in early parent-child interactions. A mate, then, sees only the perfect facade of narcissistic defense. One may seek admiration and appreciation and when it is not forthcoming feels emptiness and deflation. The other seeks understanding and acceptance and when deprived of it experiences frustration and anger. Such narcissistic collusive patterns underlie many issues—money, work, children's problems, sexual dysfunction, and so on—that on the surface appear to be the source of the marital problems. Through projective defenses it is possible to split off internalized, unacceptable impulses and feelings and hand them over to a mate who is more or less willing to accept them.

The prevailing view has been that increases in differentiation among family members bring about positive intrapsychic changes, including some resolution of past conflicts and higher levels of personality maturation. With increases in differentiation comes a greater ability to function both mentally and physically (Bowen, 1972). There is, then, an implicit assumption of a strong, "non-negotiable self," having autonomous values and living up to them in an ethical, responsible manner (Bowen, 1976). Within this paradigm, the capacity to separate the self from others corresponds with an ability to form mature relationships.

Our current cultural messages, which reflect this view, suggest that it is wise for an individual to avoid extended dependence on parents or spouse. Accordingly, separation from one's family of origin is seen as a step toward the development of a mature ability to form intimate relationships. The importance of one's independence and self-esteem is a basic tenet of our society, but it makes little sense to work toward separation and differentiation exclusively when the whole purpose of an intimate relationship is mutuality and interdependence. Partners who are free to accept and understand each other's infantile needs are also free to support each other's search for individual satisfaction. A mature desire for another to function as an extension of the self, if limited in duration and coupled with realistic expectations of reciprocity, is a normal aspect of a relationship in our culture. It is important to recognize that adults continue to have certain childlike needs. Indeed, some needs, such as the desire for empathy, affirmation and nurturance, are never fully outgrown (Kohut, 1977).

LIFELONG NEEDS FOR SELF OBJECTS

Kohut (1977) used the term "selfobject" to describe the interpersonal attunement between the emerging self of the infant and the caretaking other. The selfobject provides needed functions until the child has developed internal capacities and self structures. Furthermore, Kohut proposed a lifelong need for selfobject relatedness. Love relationships must include mutual, self-esteem-enhancing mirroring and idealization, Kohut suggested. "It is characteristic of a healthy self that it is not forced to go it alone at all costs but that it can, in emergencies, turn toward the support of selfobjects" (1971, p. 278).

"A good marriage," Kohut said, "is one in which one partner or the other rises to the challenge of providing the selfobject function that the other's temporarily impaired sense of self needs at a particular moment" (1984, p. 220). From birth to death, self-selfobject relationships form the essence of psychological life: "a move from dependence . . . to independence . . . in the psychological sphere is no more possible, let alone desirable, than a corresponding move from a life dependent on oxygen to a life independent of it in the biological sphere" (Kohut, 1984, p. 47).

In marriages that work, the partners have learned to understand and respond to each other's underlying needs in a mutual exchange without either one's feeling diminished. Each uses the other at times as an "object" for restoration, consolidation, transformation and organization of internal experience in order to maintain or regain feelings of cohesiveness.

BOUNDARIES

Boundaries define the limits of the marriage and its relationship to the outside world. There are boundaries within the self (intrapsychic process structures), boundaries between the two individuals (experiential differences), and boundaries between the couple and the environment in which they live (sociocultural limits). Within this last boundary each seeks shelter in the other from outside pressures.

Excessively rigid, impermeable boundaries inhibit growth, constrict and devitalize. Excessively flexible, diffuse boundaries permit chaos to reign and create fear of dissolution. One of the primary tasks of marriage and marriage therapy is the establishment of clear, permeable boundaries that maintain balance not only within the dyad but between the couple and the world.

A healthy relationship has boundaries that are clearly delineated and balanced. In a well-functioning relationship, partners retain their unique identities and respect each other's separateness and individuality. Boundaries are sufficiently solid, thus allowing for privacy, and sufficiently permeable to allow interpersonal communication. While each individual has a private sphere that is not shared with anyone, identity formation and identity preservation require continuing communication with others.

There are many highly functioning individuals today who feel capable of being in intimate relationships but wonder why they feel so emotionally isolated. In some cases it is the result of single-minded striving in the belief (conscious or unconscious) that each person must develop independently at all costs. Any merging or blurring of boundaries is taken as a regression to earlier, less functional kinds of relatedness. Viewing maturity only in terms of differentiation results in a loss of ability to use intimate relationships as a safe haven for regressing to dependent states in times of need or stress. Often I have heard a husband or a wife say of the other, "I don't need another child," rejecting the possibility of safe periods of regression. Paradoxically, it is through a willingness to regress temporarily that nonpathological selfobject needs may be met.

What we call enmeshment is not in itself necessarily pathological. It may be part of a tendency among intimate family members to temporarily remove the boundaries between them and experience periods of merger. Intimacy occurs when regressive needs can be met occasionally and reciprocally. When there are pathological family members who use open boundaries and the vulnerability of others to satisfy their own huge demands for attention and affirmation, then the kinds of pathological situations that are described in the family therapy literature may develop. However, the assumption that merging of boundaries between family members causes a pathological "undifferentiated family ego mass" (Bowen, 1972) must be reexamined in light of current developmental knowledge.

Undifferentiation becomes a problem when early development has left an inadequate sense of self. Then the normal wish to reexperience the comforting feeling of peaceful merger becomes entangled with the anxiety or even dread of loss of self and engulfment within the boundaries of some outside force. This kind of internal conflict causes a number of problems in intimacy, including a longing for a loving illusion of oneness and a panic-driven withdrawal from genuine relationship. Love is mixed with a fear of becoming close, feelings of dissolution, and severe anxiety about any separation, along with a fantasy of ongoing merger with the loved one. The defenses, created in response to early fears of incorporation or abandonment, may be aimed at isolating the individual from the possibility of intimacy with others or at protecting the self from the dangers that may arise in loving or being loved. The question of boundaries and their importance in the therapeutic situation is also discussed in Chapter 9.

THE MUTUAL SELF

The partners' individual behavior is shaped not only by temperament, personality characteristics and early history, but also by the *mutual self* or *joint personality* that emerges from the marital interaction. In being and acting as a unit, mates exercise an important influence over each other, whether they acknowledge it or not and whether they like it or not. Behavior patterns evolve mutually: "In this relationship, I do not cause your behavior, nor do you cause my behavior. Rather, we shape each other's behavior and, consequently, our own in a reverberating interaction." Once the pattern has evolved, it sustains itself relatively well.

In adult relationships partners may assist, complement or replace each other in specific tasks, taking responsibility for certain aspects of their joint life together. As they grow increasingly attuned to each other, the marital system develops a life force of its own, a force so strong that the inner life of one partner no longer can exist totally independently of the other's (Willi, 1982). Creation of a mutual self is based upon complementariness, an unconscious division of functions in which each partner supplies part of a set of qualities, the sum of which is a complete unit greater than the sum of its parts. Their joint personality permits the partners to recapture lost aspects of their primary object relations, which they reexperience in their involvement with each other (Dicks, 1967).

The marital system incorporates the adaptations implicit in a new social relationship and the adaptations implicit in a new emotional relationship. The former reflect, among other things, the values, beliefs, and organization of partners' families; the latter reflect, primarily, the early emotional histories of the partners themselves.

In a poorly functioning marriage, internal patterns learned early in life cause distortions in each partner's perception of the other. The inner narrative of each partner accounts, virtually completely, for the actions of the other, so that each projects on the other positive and negative fantasies that may have little to do with that person's actual motivations. In some relationships, partners assume that the other sees and wants what they themselves see and want. The couple operates unconsciously and automatically within a system of recursive rules that recirculate with frightening regularity, and no growth is possible.

ESTABLISHMENT OF A MUTUAL COMFORT ZONE

There is always a balance between the two poles of the system. At one end is the need for inclusion in the human group, the lack of which leaves a sense of cosmic psychic isolation. At the other extreme is the experience of absolute enmeshment, total transparency, "in which no single corner of potentially shareable experience can be kept private" (Stern, 1985, p. 136).

When a couple begins to live together, they establish an *emotional comfort zone*, or homeostasis. It is as if there is a thermostat that keeps the relationship from being too hot (i.e., too merged) or too cold (i.e., too distant). A couple's observable struggle to get along can camouflage the fundamental struggle of each partner to maintain the balance between separateness and connectedness necessary for individual psychic survival. These struggles are played out in the covert and overt messages spouses give each other. For some the message is, "Don't get too close or I will suffocate." For others it is, "Don't move out of emotional contact for a moment or I will feel abandoned and fear that I will die." In either case, the message is urgently and deeply felt. Depending upon the degree of disturbance, there may be a fear of both extremes: "Don't get close, but don't go away. If you withdraw emotionally I will start a fight to pull you back into my orbit because I need desperately for you to be there." Painful contact is better than none at all.

Creation of the emotional comfort zone reactivates conflicts with early significant figures (Framo, 1980, 1982). Although members of the family of origin may be long gone or reside in a distant city, they continue to live inside a person as introjects, internal representations. While a marital pair is establishing an identity as a couple, they are at the same time, on an unconscious level, recreating certain aspects of their separate inner worlds, their early relationship with their parents. Together, they recapitulate earlier relationship with their parents. Together, they recapitulate earlier conflictual experiences.

The creation of a joint mutual self gives rise to many collective fantasies, both progressive and regressive. The formation and maintenance of a marital system involves a series of small and large crises and continuous decision-making. Each partner is challenged to grow while simultaneously dealing with his or her own regressive needs. In functioning relationships, partners benefit from being able to alternate freely between roles. Roles are constantly redefined as the couple "co-evolves" to handle the challenges of life. Various problems—childbirth, loss of a job, illness, and so on—initiate changes in the positions taken by husband and wife.

MAINTENANCE OF HOMEOSTASIS

Therapists working individually with patients have often noted that as the patient improves the marriage deteriorates. Meanwhile child therapists bemoan the fact that as soon as the child improves the parents discontinue treatment, claiming that things had gotten worse instead of better. The greater the pathology, the harder the system will work to nullify the effects of therapy.

The projection of intrapsychic conflict onto others, who are then perceived and responded to accordingly, is designed to reinforce and preserve a particular level of intrapsychic functioning. This maintains an equilibrium, keeping stable either the happiness or the misery of a relationship by allowing change and movement only within a certain range. Once the limits are reached, the system returns to its original state of equilibrium, for better or worse. In pathological relationships, a number of defenses come into play to reestablish former interactional exchanges (Slipp, 1984). One way already noted is the manipulation of external reality so that it is consistent with expectations and congruent with early object relations. The responses of the other are internalized in such a way as to provide reinforcement of a dangerously tinged internal world, perhaps through perception of only those messages of the other that conform to a predetermined set of expectations.

A change in any one part of a family produces one of several possible reactions. The family may modify itself to accommodate changes in an individual member. Alternately, the forces within the family may be called into play in order to reestablish the equilibrium. If they cannot find a way to establish a new and acceptable homeostatic balance, the family system may self-destruct. A child leaves home or a relationship ends.

When people marry, subliminal agreements emerge that determine interactions. There is an early period in which the couple makes conscious and unconscious decisions about how this marriage will function. Partners become involved in issues of emotional distance-closeness, dependence-

independence, sexual availability, responsibility for relationship maintenance, relatedness to others and decisions about children. How closely the
internal representational models of the world mesh often determines the
comfort level of the relationship. When partners' values, beliefs, and cultural heritage differ widely, everything must be negotiated. That in itself does
not mean a marriage will be unhappy. When there is a history of narcissistic vulnerability, however, it interferes with the ability to discuss and compromise. Instead, differences are perceived as threatening to the cohesiveness of the self. Demands that the mate function in ways that protect the
vulnerabilities from emerging damage one or both partners. The result is a
collusive pattern that seems to be causing considerable unhappiness, but
actually serves the purpose of maintaining a fragile equilibrium for both
partners.

TRIANGULATION

When a stable system becomes filled with anxiety, the couple often brings
in a third party to counteract marital tensions (Bowen, 1976). Such
"triangulation" protects against excessive intimacy by removing opportunities for one-on-one encounters. The spouses can form an alliance against a
threatening third party. Henry and Diana become closer whenever Diana's
mother came to visit. Both could see her as a common challenge or threat,
reuniting them and pushing their own marital tensions into the background. However, Diana could also bring her mother into the conflict as
her ally. Henry, feeling betrayed, generally tried to find an ally for himself,
expanding the circle of conflict even further. As in most marital conflicts,
there was fluctuation of alternating triangles.

    As each child is born, parents whose relationship is unstable or anxiety-
producing draw the child into a new triangle. Because of this, the children's
developmental needs are not responded to, which inhibits their growth.
This perpetuates the familial pathology and predisposes the children to
have the same problems as their parents. Through formation of covert
alliances, the triangle saves the marriage partners, who are unable to tolerate the anxiety caused by their own internal or external difficulties. On the
other hand, it is not unusual for two children then to form an alliance to
protect themselves against powerful parents.

    The triangulation, then, is an understood but unstated collusion be-
tween emotionally damaged mates. In a case that I was called upon for
consultation, a couple was referred for treatment by their child's therapist.
There was a concern about the father's return to the home after serving
time in a prison and a state hospital for molesting his daughter, then 11

years old. The daughter was 16 when the mother invited her husband to return home. It became clear from the history that the mother, a frightened and inadequate woman, avoided sexual contact with her husband by offering her child in her place. The mother cut herself off from the family, informing them that from 9 to 11 p.m. she was not to be disturbed during her religious meditations. She locked herself in the bedroom that she shared with her husband, locking him out. The father took advantage of the meditation period to become involved sexually with his daughter. In family sessions with a relatively inexperienced family therapist, the couple did not focus on the destructive systemic collusion: the father's deviance and the mother's silent accommodation. The daughter's provocative and promiscuous behavior was the issue in treatment; thus she retained the scapegoat role.

Most family triangles are less tragic, but the collusive process is similar. In order to protect one or more members of the family, there is an unconscious agreement among the family members that one person will act out the pathology and save the others. The weakest member of the family is often assigned the role of being "sick."

THE FALSE SELF IN MARRIAGE

The condition that has been identified as schizoid (Fairbairn, 1954a) or as the "false self" (Winnicott, 1965, 1971) results when, without conscious awareness, a person consistently shuts out large portions of the feeling messages sent by others. Winnicott suggested that the false self develops as a caretaker of the true self, providing a protective exterior that allows a measure of privacy, a sense of integrity, and safety from any threat of annihilation through being subsumed by another. Once learned, the false self defense is carried on throughout life and acted upon in situations where threats to integrity of self and wish for love are in conflict.

Nancy, a female business executive, very successful in her career, presented such a concern to me in a rather generalized way, saying, "You know, when I was in graduate school I talked to a lot of my fellow students. We were at the top of our class, and yet we all had this same feeling that we were really fooling everyone into believing that we were successful. We worked tremendously hard to look good, but underneath it all we knew that there was no substance there." Once she shared this feeling, which seemed so embarrassing to her at first, she found it much easier to speak about the surface the world sees and about how she had worked, sometimes to the point of exhaustion, to maintain the "false picture" seen by the world.

The false self has its roots in the very early trauma of tolerating obligation and responsibility to others. This requires an awareness of what Winnicott (1971) calls "not-me" objects, accepting the other as separate from the self, with a divergent identity and needs. For some the experience is one of an emptiness within and the result is a defensive exclusion designed to protect a vulnerable self. Because they are exquisitely sensitive to failures, disappointments, and slights, those with false selves have learned to submerge feelings and put their emotional energy into developing relationships in which they can maintain an illusion of loving and being loved by others.

Such people desperately wish for a relationship, may even believe that they are in a relationship, but can accomplish only a "sense of relatedness" (Wynne, 1987) that lacks a firm base. They overlook what is really going on with the other, what the other person is truly like. They are not satisfied in their relationships and do not know what to do with partners' complaints about their inability to demonstrate emotion. Often they say that they would like to feel more emotion, but do not know how. Because they are generally desirous of maintaining their relationships, however disappointing, they often willingly, but with trepidation, enter into and continue in marital therapy in an attempt to repair whatever is wrong. Such individuals are capable of change, but do so only with great difficulty, despite their apparently earnest efforts.

Ron, a middle-aged investment banker, had to work hard to maintain a façade of success. His inner feeling was one of vacancy – an emptiness that was often "too painful to bear." Yet the world saw him as charming, the life of the party, and part of an ideal marriage. He was just at the point of leaving his wife when one of his employees, newly engaged, came to him and said that he only hoped to have a married life as wonderful as Ron's. Because of this expectation of his employee, with whom he had only a peripheral relationship, Ron did not leave.

THE FEAR OF BEING ALONE

For some there may remain throughout life a craving to fill an indefinable emptiness, which can lead at the same time to humiliation and to embarrassed denial of neediness. A person who greatly desires to be dependent and cared for may end up instead taking care of others. Such a person may, for example, encourage a partner to become dependent or ineffectual, thus assuring that the other will never leave, and that the vulnerable individual will not be abandoned.

Helen, the fourth wife of a successful attorney, sought a divorce after three years of marriage. She could not stand the way David insisted that she be near him all the time. While he had no objections to her working during the day, he expected her to be home before he got there to prepare dinner every night. That, she said, she could understand. After dinner, however, he wanted her to be in the same room with him and do whatever he was doing. He would, for example, become enraged with her if she closed her eyes while they watched television. She left him when, one evening, he interrogated her when she got up to go to the bathroom.

DAVID Where are you going?
HELEN To the bathroom.
DAVID Are you coming back?
HELEN (angrily) Will you please stop asking me that!
DAVID (hurt) Why are you so upset?

His difficulties with Helen confirmed for David that there is no way to have a loving relationship with a woman. "I give them everything—they give nothing in return." David believed that he was all-giving and terribly mistreated. In fact, a fear of being left alone, which he had carried with him all his life, permeated and ultimately destroyed all of his relationships.

This particular failure occurs in those who as infants came to expect greatly delayed and deferred responses to their needs. They become extremely upset at any sign of coming distress because they fear that relief will take an intolerably long time to arrive. Depending upon what protective defenses develop, the child may become very anxious and panicked at times when left alone, and even as an adult may feel abandoned the moment there is no warm body in the room. The husbands and wives of these individuals complain of feeling "smothered" or "strangled" by the tight hold of a frightened child in an adult's body.

WITHDRAWN MARRIAGES

A common reaction to narcissistic injury is emotional withdrawal even as the couple remains united in the eyes of others. Often couples rationalize their withdrawal from one another as preoccupation with activities that will benefit the couple or the family as a whole. Withdrawn couples show a pattern of "pseudo-mutuality." They make a strong attempt to maintain the appearance of a relationship, the illusion that they have an open, mutually understanding way of interacting, when in reality they maintain great distance between one another. What they do have in common is a shared maneuver designed to defend against pervasive feelings of meaninglessness and emptiness. There is a great determination to maintain the illusion of family unity. Any potential for growth and autonomy is squashed and sacrificed for the purpose of holding the couple or family together.

Some such couples appear at first glance to be close, caring and responsible, but the partners are overwhelmed by their obligations. These obligations justify emotional distance and withdrawal, used not to conceal but to avoid the inner rage or fragility that both recognize could come out a little too easily and damage their relationship. They also fear that intimacy will expose their fear of humiliation and proneness to fragmentation. Their emotional withdrawal is rationalized by another attachment, one that has value to the family as a whole, such as a job or civic responsibilities. They may put their attention on the children, even going so far as to pressure the children to engage in dysfunctional behavior, or the children may collude with them by adopting dysfunctional behavior, so the parents have even more of an excuse to attend to them rather than to each other.

It seems that these spouses live together only for the sake of the children or for material advantage. Behind their restrained façade, both partners are watching and trying to control each other in all their thoughts and actions. Indifferent behavior becomes a desperate defense against too much intimacy. Larry described his relationship with Gwen as being like "two porcupines ready to shoot quills at each other." They have their work, their hobbies, their sports and their exercise. She feigns ignorance when he complains that she is not there emotionally, but he recognizes that he does the same to her. When they are not fighting, they live totally separate lives. He spends most of his time on the boat in the marina, where he has a whole separate group of friends. She is busy with her bridge and charity work, which he avoids as much as possible. Since their son left for college, they hate to be near one another. They make sure to have others join them when they go out to dinner or on vacation, because they have nothing to say to each other.

Sometimes when there has been a history of narcissistic injury, partners will withdraw from each other whenever there is a danger of too much intimacy. If they allow feelings of closeness or lower their barriers, they open themselves to the heretofore unachievable wish to fill a deep well of needs. Unfortunately, they recognize that by such closeness they have exposed themselves to the possibility of massive disappointment.

RECIPROCITY OF CONSCIOUS AND UNCONSCIOUS AGREEMENTS: A CASE STUDY

All couples enter into agreements during courtship and the early part of the marriage. Many agreements tend to rigidify into particular patterns based upon undiscussed preconscious and unconscious patterns. Changes in this verbal contract may occur throughout the marriage, based upon certain events that shake up the balance of the relationship, such as the arrival of a new family member, financial strain, illness, or the loss of a job.

Michael and Barbara had a prenuptial agreement in which each independently kept all the assets they had before their marriage. Michael was a successful real estate broker and Barbara worked as a beautician. They bought a home together but the down payment came from the sale of one of Michael's real estate investments. They signed an additional contract stating that half of the proceeds from the eventual sale of the house would be Barbara's or would be put into a larger home to be owned by them jointly. Their plan was to buy a larger home when they had children. They also had a verbal agreement that they would wait two years before having a baby. At that point Barbara was to give up working and take full-time charge of the home. Until that time, he agreed to share certain specific household tasks.

Unfortunately, the real estate market took a downturn and Michael's business and their home lost much of its value. Barbara began to question whether she wanted to put in the effort of improving a home that was, in fact, not hers. In addition, she was not sure that their finances were secure enough for her to give up work to have a baby. She was feeling a need to protect her financial future. Michael could not understand this. He did not doubt his ability to support a wife and child and wondered why Barbara, if she intended to remain married to him, felt a need for her own income. What he now wanted was to put all of his energies into his career in order to make up for some of his losses, while Barbara stayed home and had the baby as agreed. She suggested that they talk it over with a counselor, as she was uncomfortable with the situation but not certain what to do.

Michael and Barbara decided to have a child with the stipulation that Barbara would return to work within a few months and Michael would assist with childcare and housework. When the baby was six months old, Michael's company was forced into bankruptcy and Michael took a job in a large real estate firm. He worked long hours and came home tired. Their income was much more limited than it had been when they married, but with some belt tightening they were largely able to maintain their standard of living. At that point, Michael suggested that Barbara give up her job and take charge of the home, as he could not share the responsibilities at home and make a success of his new job. He felt that he could make so much more than she did that it would be best if he put in his time into supporting the family and paying off debts incurred in his past business, while she took care of everything in the home. Barbara agreed to this. However, the marriage soon deteriorated into a round of complaints by each to and about the other. The relationship was affected by unconscious and unstated factors which were, therefore, inaccessible to them for use in reaching any agreement.

Michael was born in 1942; Barbara in 1951. The age difference was less a factor than the generational difference. He was almost an adult when the feminist movement came into full swing; the rebellion of the 1960s was taking place while he was serving in Vietnam. While Michael repeatedly said, "I'm no male chauvinist," he found it very hard to let go of the values instilled by his family. He believed that it was up to a man to be responsible for his family and felt that he lost status in his wife's eyes by putting her in a position where she had to work. He also hated housework and found himself resenting his wife every time he had to help with the laundry or the dishes. He said that he enjoyed being with the baby and would help with that, but Barbara commented that he returned the baby to her every time the diapers had to be changed.

Barbara was 29 years old when she married, had traveled extensively, and loved the freedom of being independent as much as she feared remaining single. As a full-time housewife and mother she was feeling increasingly restrained and claustrophobic. She was also angry at Michael for his financial difficulties but did not want to sound like a spoiled "princess." She did not complain verbally, but evened things out by not doing the little extra things that had always pleased him. She no longer made plans for the weekend with other couples, she suggested that he balance the checkbook, she fell asleep when they were together watching television and was too tired for sex.

Since Barbara was always overtly compliant, Michael did not know what to do with the resentment and anger he felt when it seemed that Barbara was not carrying her share of the burden in the marriage while he worked so hard to improve their situation. He found it increasingly frustrating to go home and began to stay later and later at work. The result was that he had success at work but had a wife who felt very neglected. Each was failing the other without quite knowing why or what to do about it.

When Michael and Barbara met, each had an idealized picture of the other. He was older, wiser, a father figure to make up for Barbara's own father, who vanished from her life when she was six years old and her parents got divorced. She had always imagined that, if she had had an opportunity to show her father how much she loved him, he would not have abandoned them. She felt extraordinarily lucky that such a wonderful man as Michael wanted to marry her and was determined to do everything necessary to make Michael stay with her forever. She had never felt so alive and energetic as when they first met.

Michael, too, remembered with fondness their early times together. After two disastrous marriages, here, finally, he felt that he had found a perfect match. When they were together it felt as though they were united, "one body, one mind," he explained. He felt he could achieve anything with "her by my side." At times he still felt that, but it was because of feedback from others rather than from her. Now she often seemed so depressed and withdrawn that he had to avoid her so as not to be dragged down. She was just never there anymore when he needed her.

Both felt that their needs were not being met. Each felt neglected in an area of vulnerability. Each experienced narcissistic injury and put up a protective shield. The way that each one protected a vulnerable self resulted in injury to the other. The lack of clear awareness of the cause of the hurt and the anticipation of further hurt feelings kept them from discussing their problems with each other. They retaliated for real and imagined hurts increasingly at preconscious or unconscious levels.

In a loving relationship, there is an unstated agreement that no one will misuse information about things that can throw the other into a state of extreme fear, pain, fragmentation, or violent acting-out. The more damaged the psyche, the more sensitive the individual is to such injury, but there are few indeed who can withstand the experience of being psychically invaded or attacked without ever retaliating or withdrawing emotionally. Unconscious defenses take many forms and have serious effects on the ability to maintain relationships.

Michael and Barbara argued over apparently inconsequential matters. He became angry when he saw her putting the new packages of frozen hamburger meat into the freezer in the front of the packages bought earlier. When he became angry at her she cried. When she cried he became enraged, yelling that she just wanted to feel sorry for herself and would never listen to what he told her. When he asked her questions about why she behaved in ways that were clearly not logical, she became even more illogical, talking about other things to change the subject.

When discussing this in therapy, Barbara recognized that she argued in a roundabout way, avoiding answering his questions because they felt like a trap to her. She always ended up feeling stupid and incompetent. Ultimately resorting to arguing her way, he got even more upset than she did and became no more competent than she at that point. Michael made a conscious decision to remain logical and to discuss differences clearly, but each time an argument began he became enraged again.

Michael and Barbara had severe ongoing difficulty in their relationship for a long time after they entered therapy. When they began, the future of their marriage seemed very precarious. As I often have seen, however, it is very difficult to predict from an initial consultation whether a couple will choose to fight to overcome the odds against them and to make their marriage work, or will decide to divorce. Barbara and Michael continued in conjoint therapy for two years, declining recommendations that they consider individual therapy or group therapy as well. They terminated marital therapy a year before this writing and are still married. When I call to make follow-up contacts, they report that the most severe arguments rarely occur now. Barbara called me a few months ago to report the birth of their second child. While their marriage still has many unresolved issues, Barbara reported, "he listens to me now . . . ," "he understands that when I tell him something is important to me, it really is important." "Of course," she added, "I am very careful not to say too many things are important; then he listens to me when I do insist on something." Many would find such a relationship intolerable. Michael and Barbara did not ask me if I considered theirs a "good enough" marriage. They appear to be succeeding in making their interactional pattern work to a degree tolerable to them.

THE HEALING NATURE OF A FUNCTIONAL RELATIONSHIP

Sometimes two people with serious vulnerabilities to injury succeed in serving in a capacity for each other that promotes the well-being of both. In a loving relationship it is possible for the partners to develop a mutual interplay and reciprocity that, while imperfect and subject to the usual stresses of living together, provides a reparative function. Each legitimizes his or her own residue of child-like needs by caring for the other. They become more tolerant of each other's needs and of their own. Some needs are gratified, others remain partially unmet without causing damaged feelings. When partners hear and are responsive to the other's internal world, as a couple they may overcome great adversity. Many families overcome the illness and death of a child or severe financial difficulties. It is not the stress of life but the ability to see the relationship as a haven in a difficult world that defines marital satisfaction.

I saw two couples in marital therapy, each of whom had an oldest son diagnosed as autistic. The first couple ended up divorcing and the wife blamed the child for the breakdown of a good relationship. The second couple searched out other parents of autistic children, developed an educational program, and found ways to raise funds for research on autism. They said that their life was much more difficult than they had anticipated, that the marriage had been rocky at points, but that they had become a support system for each other. In a follow-up contact several years later, this couple reported that they felt their marriage had become stronger as a result of their problems with their son.

Sometimes a functional relationship can have healing effects. Greg and Jessica were both physically abused as children—he by a schizophrenic mother, she by her stepfather. Jessica's explanation to herself and to her therapist of her success as an adult is that she has absolute confidence that Greg accepts her, even when she hates herself. The confirmation that she gets consistently from Greg has slowly given her the confidence to try her skills in the world outside. Her talent as an artist, an ability she barely knew that she had, has grown into a successful career. In turn, she says that she would never say or do anything to injure his self-esteem. She believes that she knows what he needs, just as he understands her needs. Alone she felt anxious and withdrawn. Together, she says, "we can conquer the world."

Alan and Adelle each come from families that were far from ideally nurturing. Alan's mother died when he was $2^1/2$. His father had a series of girlfriends, each of whom were kind to Alan and his older sister, perhaps in hopes of marrying their father. But the father, who had been deeply affected by the serious illness and death of his wife, reacted by never allowing himself to invest fully in another relationship. He spent much of his time as a salesman, traveling throughout the country, while his children went to live with various relatives for periods of three to six months at a time.

Adelle grew up in a united lower-middle-class family in which her parents were obsessed with becoming upper-middle-class through working long hours in a small family business. Their emotional energies were invested mainly in an older son, who was the family's pride and joy. Adelle felt unlovable and unloved throughout her growing up years. She used very little of her talents and inner resources until she met Alan.

Through their union each expected to have the emptiness filled and insecurities alleviated. He looked to her to replace the loving mother who would love and cherish him and would never leave or abandon him. She looked to Alan to be the idealized father who would both take care of her when she felt weak or insecure and have faith in her abilities to accomplish anything that she set out to do—a faith that she lacked within herself. Their marriage was clearly working for each of them. They were two peas in a pod.

What seems clear is that early vulnerability and a history of narcissistic failure alone do not cause unhappy marriages. Nor is it simply that partners select each other because they are at a similar developmental level (Dicks, 1967; Giovacchini, 1965), in order to recreate and perpetuate unhappy early relationships. Rather, partners tend to choose each other with the unconscious hope of repeating what was good and repairing what felt bad or lacking in earlier primary interactions.

ROMANTIC LOVE

The state of being in love enhances the self through the process of fusion and idealization. For a time two become one; it feels timeless and forever. Idealization is a normal part of falling in love, but can turn into a pathological defense when partners feel they must repress hostile feelings toward one another, or demand that there be a perfect merger of thought and feelings to maintain their love.

"There is a driving passion in new love which overcomes reason, logic, and the wish to be a separate autonomous person" (Lang, 1985). Lovers find in the reflection of each other's gaze a sense of being enjoyed, appreciated, affirmed, special, unique, and loved. Regression to childlike states and feelings is a common experience of new lovers. Notice how lovers at the height of romantic passion use "baby talk" and childlike diminutive names with each other. They join together emotionally and intertwine physically, as though trying to destroy any boundary between them. Words are not necessary.

Lovers feel transformed by the spark that passes between them. Each functions as a "signifier of transformation." " . . . [T]he quest is not to possess . . . rather the object is pursued in order to surrender to it as a medium that alters the self" (Bollas, 1987, p. 3). Being with the loved one is experienced as a transformation of the self; this metamorphosis is not simply an illusion. When we observe someone newly in love, the joy, aliveness, and vigor are readily apparent. Two people in love share a common fantasy. Each sees the other as the "special someone" to whom he will be totally devoted and who, in turn, will be totally devoted to him. A state of exultation prevails that enhances the value of each for the other. "A person in love may well overvalue the object of his ardor but in no way diminishes himself. . . . The love object of the narcissist is a twofold mirror of himself, and he may well belittle himself in order to accentuate the lofty grandeur of his own reflection . . . even the earthworm in love with the star basks in the reflection of the star's brilliance" (Grunberger, 1971, pp. 4–5).

A fused attachment begins at the time partners first "fall in love." In the passion of a new love, the idealization process begins and both experience themselves as whole and loved. Each feels beautiful when reflected in the shining light of the idealized other. As they share themselves with each other, the love deepens. Both feel that the other knows and reflects back their most inner selves, their fears, vulnerabilities, wishes, and grand plans for the future. Each feels heard, understood, and responded to. Each for a time experiences being perfectly mirrored by an ideal other. During this time there is a feeling of being fulfilled; for the moment there is no awareness of anything lacking in self or in other. Together they are one, and the one is whole.

BEYOND THE ILLUSION

After the idealized fusion of romantic love, partners begin the unconscious work of determining what they can expect in the way of emotional fulfillment. Much of that is through the sending and receiving of messages at a preverbal level. Body motions, including touching, posture, the sound of the voice, and eye contact, are the primary language of intimate love relationships. "Will you love me if you know me?" is the question asked repeatedly. "How much can I show of me and still be accepted by you? Can I let you know when I am scared? When I am weak? When I feel crazy? Can I tell you that I am insecure about losing my job? Or will you fall apart with your own anxiety? Can you accept the reality of what I am attempting to tell you about my inner self? Will you simply translate what I tell you into your own expectations, wishes, and thoughts about how people are or how they should be?"

The desire for another who functions as an unconditional mirror, the tendency to adore another as an ideal, the need for an understanding alter-ego and the wish for the other to accept and contain anxiety-arousing and fearful feelings are not unrealistic to the extent that they are limited in duration and are coupled with reasonable expectations of reciprocity. If marriage partners recognize, consciously or unconsciously, that some child-like needs are never fully outgrown, but can be satisfied and enjoyed, they exchange the role of meeting selfobject needs for each other without feeling diminished.

In the intimacy of marriage or a serious relationship, difficulties arise, over the long run, when partners fail to accept undisclosed, thinly veiled aspects of each other. When these boundaries are open and vulnerabilities exposed, one's wish is to be truly known and still loved. When love is not forthcoming or there is a feeling of being judged and shamed, defenses go up to protect the vulnerable self. There is a need to exert active control over negative aspects of the self in such a way as to evade feelings of hopelessness, fragmentation, or despair.

When partners feel safe to drop their shields with each other, they no longer need to put energy into defenses. Instead they have the freedom to explore themselves, to grow and test out changes. As this occurs they have more to share with each other and there is more energy and fulfillment in the relationship. They lose the fear that what will spontaneously emerge is dangerous, damaging, or destructive to themselves, others, or the relationship. Their experience in the relationship has made them feel reassured that their words will not later come back as accusations or negative judgments of themselves. The capacity to read within oneself what someone else is trying to project elsewhere provides the means for empathic understanding—to stand in the shoes of another.

We see, then, several aspects of narcissism in relationships. There is the wish for merger that is seen in its most obvious and culturally acceptable form in the process of falling in love. There is the normal need for times of regression to dependence and neediness in which the mate functions in ways that affirm the self. There is also the need of the narcissistically vulnerable to sustain a precarious self that is constantly in danger of fragmentation by having another present at all times to serve certain self-enhancing functions. The varying aspects of narcissism will be discussed in more detail in Chapter 3. Either partner may be called upon to respond in this way some of the time or all of the time, depending upon the degree of health or vulnerability in each, and the state of the relationship. In a mature relationship either mate may call upon the other to provide needed functions. At the same time each understands that the other has a right to decide that his or her own needs are greater at that point, and can tolerate not getting the wished-for response. This occurs when the couple system is built upon mutual respect and trust; although emotional needs are not immediately met, they do not result in fear of fragmentation or a rapid buildup of preexisting defenses against the loss of a cohesive self. Thus a functioning marriage contributes to the stability and well-being of each partner.

CHAPTER 3

The Narcissistic Continuum

Many people consider narcissism to be the enemy of intimate relationships. I do not. Narcissism and intimacy are not necessarily conflicting terms. To many, "narcissist" denotes an abiding and pathological self-centeredness or even a discrete psychopathological disorder. I contend that narcissism is not in itself an illness, but an aspect of relatedness in which the principal focus is on the self and its pressing needs. This chapter will look at narcissism as a continuum from archaic to mature forms.

In mature narcissism lies the ability to combine talents and skills with ambitions to accomplish important life goals. Romantic love includes narcissistic components; parenting, too, includes the narcissistic investment in childrearing, and often an idealized vision of the child as a container of future hopes and aspirations. Mentoring relationships in adulthood also include aspects of idealization on the receiver's side and the mentor's pleasure of sharing achievements and deriving esteem and admiration.

On the other hand, persons with more archaic forms of narcissism are characterized by exquisite sensitivity to psychic injury, great anxiety, fear of being hurt or humiliated and defensive measures that affect relationships to various degrees. When there is early damage to the structure of the developing self or to the development of identity, impairment can be carried throughout life. There is a lifelong need for particular responses from others that sometimes is seen as a totally self-centered focus. Unless later resources are available that enable the person to proceed past an inhibited development, the person may be prone to relationship problems and to behavioral or psychological disorders.

In this chapter the range of narcissistic vulnerability will be considered, from normal idealization and romance at the higher level to severe early narcissistic damage and its effect on relationships at the most archaic levels. I will introduce and describe a diagram that illustrates the internal events and experiences that cause regressions in stressful situations. After a look at the transient narcissistic states experienced at times by everyone, I will illustrate narcissistic manifestations in some case histories.

Grunberger (1979) calls "narcissism" the desire to recapture paradise lost. It is a unique and privileged state of existence, the feeling of uniqueness, wholeness, and omnipotence that was a reality only before birth. In the normal narcissism of the adult, there remains a pride derived from the illusion of uniqueness and a memory of feeling complete and whole. Narcissistic feelings reemerge when the self receives highly validating feedback from another or many others. When there is a history of narcissistic failure or injury, a pathological state may arise in which there is a turning to others for a reparative experience, in a desperate longing for fusion and mirroring, for idealized love and romance. This is also an attempt to heal the vulnerability caused by the frustrations of early life. This need is validated and encouraged by the myth of the self above all others, in our current "culture of narcissism."

Far from being unable to coexist with others, those who are narcissistically vulnerable need others excessively, to provide many self-enhancing functions. One of the most basic needs is the mirroring and affirmation that gives reassurance of being understood and loved for oneself. Idealization augments the self through identification with someone powerful and revives grandiose infantile fantasies that can bolster self-esteem during times of stress. A major means of compensating for low self-esteem is attachment to an idealized other. By selecting images of the self to fuse with the other, an individual can participate in that "perfect" other. Modeling oneself on an idealized other makes it possible to pursue otherwise unacceptably high goals without fear or guilt.

LOVE AND IDEALIZATION

A new love in many ways resembles the very earliest object relationships. In the reflection of the other's gaze a lover finds a sense of being appreciated, affirmed, and uniquely loved. The "child" in the adult will tend to replay any traumas or chronic disappointments he or she experienced in early life as part of an intimate relationship. The "child" hopes, often in vain, that a relationship with "that special someone" can repair archaic damage. A narcissistically vulnerable person tends to look for another with whom to identify. By identification, there is a hope to acquire the kind of power and strength that the other represents. For some the wish is to shine in the reflected glory of a perfect other. This idealized one is expected to remain close and consistently loving.

The belief in the perfect "oneness" that occurs in the process of new love is exemplified by Lydia, a 19-year-old airline stewardess madly in love and determined to marry despite the objections of her family. "We want to get married now," she purred, referring to her relationship with Charlie, her 42-year-old, four-times-divorced fiancé. She protested, "I don't care what other people say about our backgrounds being so different, or what happened with his other wives. You don't understand; we're *in love*. And as long as we're in love, we will be married." She added, "If it doesn't work out, we can get a divorce, but I know it will be perfect." In response to her parents' arguments that she should wait for a while until she knows him better, Lydia protested, "I know he will change for me. We're so good for each other. Only with him do I feel really alive." The fact that these are contradictory statements has little meaning for Lydia. The illusion of oneness is a repetition of an early narcissistic fantasy and exists outside the ability to distinguish contradictory ideas.

The fantasy does not last. The honeymoon is over whenever the lovers realize that they are indeed separate beings, each with individual needs and desires, which sometimes conflict. The desire to merge with one another forever impinges on the alternate desire for autonomy. Just as the infant learns that the mother is separate, and just as the child must come to terms with the reality of separateness, the illusion of merger with the loved one must give way to the recognition of the independence and separate reality of the other.

As the reality of limitations sets in, the pattern of the marriage develops and changes. The individual may expect a loving, nurturing relationship in which the partner alters his responses and even the environment in order to meet changing needs. Alternatively, the partner, unable to maintain the illusion of oneness, may be viewed with anxiety or mistrust. Defenses are built up based upon expectations of sudden withdrawal or expected failure to provide for important needs.

THE MYTH OF NARCISSUS AND
THE REALITY OF NARCISSISM

The mythical Narcissus loved himself too much. He fell in love with his reflection in a pool of water and became so enamored with what he saw that he failed to hear the endlessly repeated words of the nymph Echo, who loved him. In his own reflection he discovered a perfect other who made him feel forever whole, while soon there was nothing left of Echo but a whisper. In other versions of this myth, Narcissus was a surviving twin; the lost twin was a female whom he thought he had rediscovered in the reflected image in the pool (Bergmann, 1987).

Narcissus, of course, was entranced not by himself but by his mirror image, a perfect copy of his every nuance and movement. Unable to draw his attention away from his reflection, Narcissus was ignorant not only of Echo, but also of his own possibilities. It is this total absorption of the self that causes a distorted world view. Preconceived images of self and other are superimposed on events and responded to with the certainty that this imagined configuration of the world is the only correct interpretation. This is what makes the relationships of the modern Narcissus so problematic. These internal experiences are the precursors of narcissistic vulnerability. Regressions to earlier narcissistic states may cause or, alternatively, result from unhappy relationships. The tendency toward repetition of the first object relations in all later relationships is seen in the transference relationships that develop both in psychotherapeutic settings and in the intimacy of love relationships. An awareness of the interactional patterns that occur repeatedly between intimate partners and among family members leads to a better understanding of the expectations and disappointments that may affect love relationships.

THE NEED FOR RELATIONSHIPS

Two variables influence the course of all intimate relationships. On one hand, there is a sense of separateness and autonomy, a freedom of action. On the other hand is the universal desire for an occasional regression to a state of "symbiotic fusion"—perfect understanding by a loving other (Shor and Sanville, 1978; Horner, 1986). Finding an acceptable balance between these two desires is the dilemma of love relationships.

Despite our modern focus on the development of autonomy and individuality, there is no way to separate the self from its interrelatedness with others, because, as Tustin writes, "The sense of self and of individual identity is dependent on relationships with other people" (1987, p. 44). Relationships *do* matter. They are desperately important to our mental health, our physical well-being, our very survival. "There is no escape from a person's involvement with people, hate, love, and seeming indifference being but aspects of the entanglement" (Will, 1987, pp. 256–257). The infant cut off from human touch, even when well fed, fails to thrive; the bereft widower who dies within days or weeks of his wife's death is a reminder that the essential state of human existence is one of togetherness. Achievement of a basic sense of human connectedness is the starting point, not a later aspect of, the normal developmental process.

Mental health requires an equilibrium of relatedness—between parent and child, husband and wife, and in intimate friendships—a mutuality in which the focus on the self is balanced by recognition of another as a separate, autonomous self. Genuine mutuality tolerates a divergence of interests and thrives upon the recognition of differences between the self and others (Wynne, Ryckoff, Day, and Hirsch, 1958; Wynne, 1987). Pathological states occur when attention is riveted on the needs of the self, resulting in a loss of mutuality, either a withdrawn isolation or a "pseudomutual" appearance of relationship without true recognition of the other.

Sometimes the attempts to shore up a threatened self-image results in a distortion of the reality of the other as a separate person. The longing for a relationship combined with a narcissistic inability to tolerate "otherness" impedes the ability to experience life fully. Under such circumstances, relationships that appear objectively to be successful are experienced subjectively as empty and boring. Many marriages today are terminated for exactly that reason.

Relationships that work include some freedom for both partners to regress to child-like dependent states. The desire for another who functions as an unconditional mirror and the tendency to adore another as an ideal are not unrealistic to the extent that they are limited in duration and are coupled with reasonable expectations of reciprocity. If marriage partners recognize, consciously or unconsciously, that they continue to have at times certain childlike needs, that indeed some needs are never fully out-grown but can be satisfied and enjoyed, they exchange roles of meeting what Kohut (1977) described as "selfobject" needs for each other without either feeling diminished.

Couples who have relationship problems, but do not have a history of severe narcissistic injury, may resolve differences through compromise, problem-solving, improved communication, or through acknowledgment, acceptance, and negotiation of some basic differences. When there is a prior history of narcissistic vulnerability and failure of the other to provide necessary emotional supplies, the result is that small arguments may cause an experience of fragmentation or emotional destruction—a loss of ability to think clearly and a reaction of either rage or total withdrawal.

Narcissistic disorders include those areas of vulnerability that, in times of psychic upheaval or emotional injury, cause a loss of cohesiveness and feelings of fragmentation. Ideally the core self responds to stress with adaptations that permit endurance over time and maintenance of an experience of cohesive wholeness. If narcissistic injuries and subsequent vulnerabilities are prominent, there is a recurrent tendency to protect oneself. This is done by regression to interpersonal interchanges that recapitulate early life experiences in a selfobject relationship.

SELFOBJECTS—NORMAL AND PATHOLOGICAL

The term "selfobject" as applied to the marital relationship refers to the use of another as a vehicle for maintaining, restoring, or consolidating the internal experience of the self. Commonly expected selfobject functions include affirmation, admiration, and constant responsiveness to confirm feelings of grandiosity or to meet other self-enhancing needs. For some it is the wish to shine in the reflected splendor of a perfect other. As long as the other remains close and consistently loving, expectations for a mutually fulfilling relationship may be met. Problems develop when one partner chooses to grow in another direction or withdraws for some other reason. The disappointment and defenses that emerge may cause a rapid downward spiraling of the relationship.

Pathology may exist when there is a desperate need for the presence of the other or an urge to mold the other into an extension of oneself. There is a desire to discard boundaries while at the same time there is an anxiety about being absorbed into the other's being. One partner constantly complains about the lack of closeness and the other complains about the feeling of intrusion. At other times they may reverse these roles. Partners complain about each other, "She's always on the telephone with her mother or her friends when I am at home at night." Alternatively, "He sits at the breakfast table reading the newspaper and never even talks to me." When there are unresolved narcissistic needs, issues around closeness and distance become an ongoing problem in the relationship.

THE NARCISSISTIC CONTINUUM

Each of us functions with a core of narcissistic, self-focused views of the world. What we think of as "truths" are actually personal truths seen through a filter of early memories one built on another, layer upon layer like nested Russian dolls. The forms and structures of who we are develop early through messages instilled in the family and the culture into which we are born. The more the lens becomes deformed or distorted by early experience, the greater the narcissistic vulnerability.

The diagram in Figure 3.1 guides my exposition of narcissistic vulnerability and its effects on relationships. Throughout this book I refer to relationships that occur along a continuum which has three basic levels of self-other development: a level of mature narcissism, a transitional level which is intermediate in functioning, and an archaic level. Along the way I will describe the origins of pathology and the kind of responses to be expected from persons functioning at each level.

Reading horizontally on the diagram we see characterizations of different aspects of the functioning of individuals when their narcissistic organization is at each of the levels. I describe the internal experience of the self, stability or permeability of boundaries, object relations, types of affectual and emotional reactions, primary anxieties and the defensive measures that reflect certain specific developmental levels.

Everyone functions at various levels along the horizontal and vertical at different times, depending upon the vicissitudes and changing circumstances of life events and relationships. In situations of high stress, physical or emotional deprivation, or experiences that cause shame or humiliation, even a generally highly functioning person will regress to lower levels. Some who are extremely damaged and have had a long history of narcissistic injury may relate constantly at the more archaic narcissistic levels.

At level 3, the highest level examined, the person is generally functioning with a neurotic core, an ability to combine affect, emotion and cognition, and a recognition of the reality of self and other. There are regulating

Level	Internal Experience of Self	Boundaries	Object Relations	Primary Anxieties	Emotional System	Primary Defenses *
Level 3 Mature narcissistic states Cohesive structures	Verbal self Subjective self	Firm and flexible boundaries	Object constancy Awareness of self and other	Oedipal anxiety Castration fears Fear of injury to parts of the body	Feeling states plus thinking (cognitive awareness of emotion)	Rationalization Intellectualization Reaction Formation Sublimation (Neurotic defenses)
Level 2 Intermediate narcissistic states Transitional structures	Core self	Unstable boundaries	Impermanence of objects Use of transitional objects	Predominant concerns around identity	Emotional states Wide fluctuations of affect and emotions	Denial Isolation Undoing Splitting Projective identification Omnipotence (Borderline defenses)
Level 1 Primitive narcissistic states Archaic structures	Emergent self	Lack of self/other boundaries	Failure of object constancy Abandonment fears Illusion of omnipotent control	Survival fears Anxieties concerning existence	Affective states	Disavowal Grandiosity Halucinatory fantasy (Psychotic defenses)
Pre-Narcissistic		Autistic Border	Sense of self	has not yet	emerged	

* Defenses are part of normal development early in life. When exhibited by adults the characteristic use of certain clusters of defenses is associated with psychotic, borderline, and neurotic pathological states.

FIGURE 3.1

The Narcissistic Continuum

structures that maintain self-cohesion, a variety of ongoing functional relationships and boundaries that allow for independence and autonomy as
well as times of merger. Defenses at this level include repression, rationalization, intellectualization, reaction formation, and sublimation.

Level 2, the intermediate level of narcissistic states, is often the characteristic level of functioning for those who are at the higher state of borderline
personality organization (Kernberg, 1975). Those with narcissistic personality disorders operate at this level most of the time. Aspects of a core self
have developed and there is awareness of others, but object constancy has
not been achieved and unstable boundaries predominate. The adult who, in
times of stress, regresses to this level may be subject to fluctuating states of
joy and rage. Common defenses utilized in relationships include denial,
isolation, undoing, splitting, projective identification and grandiose demandingness.

Level 1 functioning is sometimes seen in regressions or fixations related
to borderline psychotic states in which primitive defenses are characteristic.
Although the emergent self of the newborn baby is predisposed to relatedness with the environment, there is a lack of awareness of self-other boundaries. In normal development, the child very soon after birth emerges from
any undifferentiated or autistic experience that may have existed and enters
the world of self and others. The infant responds affectively but not yet
cognitively to pleasurable and unpleasurable experience and is stimulated by
interaction with the caretaking environment. At this point, age-appropriate
structures of the self and defenses are rudimentary. It is only when they
inappropriately reemerge later in life that they are pathological. Primary
defenses at the archaic level are disavowal, omnipotence, and hallucinatory
fantasy.

Relationships with parents orient children to have certain expectations
about the way others will act and about how to respond. Sometimes the
needs of the infant and the responsiveness of the caretaker are not adequately synchronized. Chapter 4 describes how this occurs and the importance
of these early bonds to later development. Early failures cause the infant to
defend against the experience of pain in interpersonal interactions, placing a
negative cast upon subsequent developmental tasks. As people who cannot
trust others grow into adulthood, they may seek in intimate relationships
an experience that is a substitute for what is missing or that is reparative of
deep psychological wounds. The search for that perfectly attuned other
and the eruption of archaic ways of responding may undermine relationships and spread to all phases of life. The partners of those with narcissistic
vulnerabilities cannot help but become aware that something has gone

amiss, but do not always understand what part they play in the difficulties. Something akin to self-absorption keeps each uninvolved with the needs of the other except on a superficial level.

At a more pathological level, the lower border of level 1, is the autistic-psychotic experience in which the life forces are not strong enough to promote the infant into the world of reality. When earliest life events and/or constitutional deficiencies result in thwarted interactions or impediments to normal maternal bonding, the potential for development is hindered. Autistic or primitive narcissistic affectual states, boundaries, and defenses can become the primary mode of functioning. Some adults who generally function at higher levels may at times revert to a primitive autistic core. When this occurs it is frightening to them and is denied as soon as they can "pull themselves together."

People vary in how intense their feelings of vulnerability can become and in how they handle those feelings. Many narcissistically vulnerable individuals lack the ability to feel diverse emotions. They present a pseudo-sophistication to the world, but inside they experience emptiness, lethargy, or self-hate. Because they are exquisitely sensitive to failures, disappointments, and slights, they have learned to submerge feelings and put their emotional energy into developing relationships in which they can maintain an illusion of loving and being loved by others.

Since the phenomena that result from disturbances in the narcissistic investment of the self give rise to such a wide spectrum of psychic ills, we might wonder whether there are any pathologies in which narcissistic factors do not play a role. Where early experiences have left a residue of unfinished developmental tasks, there is likely to be some degree of pathology in adult relationships. The question of the extent to which phase-related developmental failures are the basis of specific pathological conditions of later life have been covered in other works (Grotstein, Solomon, and Lang, 1987). While this issue is not within the scope of this book, it is important to reiterate that when adults undergo stressful life situations they tend to regress to levels of functioning that were appropriate at earlier life stages.

The greater the vulnerability, the more the defense system will work to maintain the situation of the individual and to nullify the effects of change. Pathological regression to earlier modes of interacting limits choices, as so much that occurs in intimate relationships, threatens to open old needs and wounds. At the extremes of narcissistic vulnerability, there is a fear of fragmentation and disintegration or, alternatively, inner emptiness and deadness.

NARCISSISTIC STRUCTURES IN RELATIONSHIPS

There have been a number of well described attempts to equate various diagnostic categories in adulthood with phase-specific early developmental levels (Masterson, 1981; Rinsley, 1982). Johnson (1987) provides additional understanding of narcissism in explicit categories of psychotic, borderline, and narcissistic-style disorders. There appear to be some recognizable qualities in adults that have been observed and hypothesized to relate directly to specific early developmental phases.

At the same time we must recognize that observed pathological reactions have a basis in the relational context in which they occur. The relationships between family members are often the source of painful emotional experiences and defensive maneuvers. Before labeling unhappy marriages as being caused by the destructiveness or pathology of one mate, we must examine the behavior in relation to the context in which it emerges. While early development makes some people more prone to regressions and pathological defenses, the emergence of these reactions is caused by specific interactions with others. At the same time the degree of early damage may cause narcissistically vulnerable people to misread or misunderstand the interaction with others, thus, they are more easily provoked to defensive reactions.

With this caution I will describe some of the more pathological patterns that seem to have precursors in early developmental issues. A person whose characteristic mode of functioning is at level 1 appears subject to unstable interpersonal relationships, intense shifts in affect, attitude and behavior, lack of control of impulses and a lack of tolerance for being alone. In comparison to those whose functioning includes higher level emotional and defensive reactions, those who utilize borderline defenses (level 2) have a "less reliably constituted self with less reliable relationships with reality and less reliable self-other boundaries" (Johnson, 1987, p. 89). There is a tendency to utilize selfobjects to fulfill the function of containing overwhelming feelings. When boundaries are blurred, it is possible to assume not only that others are carriers of cast-off, unacceptable feelings, but also that those feelings in the other are destructive and must be guarded against.

Upon encountering stressful situations, the fragilely constituted and profoundly arrested self at the lower end of the borderline position of the continuum attempts to encourage—even demand—an unreal dissolution of boundaries. Where such defenses are predominant, the person may seek to merge with a source of idealized strength and calmness in order to compensate for a lack of truly independent self who can assert, "I am. I believe." What is continually expressed is, "I want, I deserve, I have rights, I get hurt," and "I get revenge on those whom I experience as hurting me." There are no shades of gray. Ambiguity or ambivalence is frightening to the borderline narcissist.

Those with a more controlled narcissistic relatedness have underlying feelings of grandiosity and entitlement, but consciously avoid such expectations. Narcissistic, archaic demands are walled off behind a facade of perfectionism and successful functioning. The "false self" (Winnicott, 1958) experiences emptiness, symptomatic interference, and limited joy, sometimes compensating with a heightened awareness of duty and obligations to others.

Under pressure of narcissistic injury, attack on the grandiose self, or lack of empathic response and affirmation, the person who functions within the range of a normal or neurotic narcissistic style will most likely seem pensive and withdrawn, while the person with the more borderline defensive structure will fragment, become fearful of feelings of disintegration, and develop defensive patterns that wreak havoc in their functioning and relationships.

INTERACTIONS ACROSS THE CONTINUUM

The following is a relatively common scenario that often occurs in relationships. To help understand how real problems may lead to narcissistic injury and marital disharmony, I will draw from a variety of situations some reactions that illustrate the narcissistic continuum at work.

Martha is a sales representative for a cosmetic company and is generally home earlier than Harry. Tonight she has cooked a special dinner for Harry because it is the anniversary of the day that they met. Meanwhile, the boss has given Harry, an engineer, an extra project with a "deadline of yesterday." Harry, immersed in his work, has forgotten to call home and did not recall that this was a special day to his wife. Martha is angry because dinner is ruined long before Harry walks in the door.

Now, if Harry and Martha are both operating on what could be termed the level of mature narcissistic functioning (level 3), so that they are able to recognize each other as having separate needs, the scenario might go something like this: Harry is met by a barrage of complaints as he walks through the door. Although he is upset by Martha's rage, he realizes that she has a right to be upset. Both are unhappy. Martha soon gets over her anger and is able to impress upon Harry that she would really like him to call if he is going to be late. Harry admits that Martha is right and promises to call. However, he explains to her that he is hoping for a promotion and that there are many contenders for the opening. He really wants the job so he will be coming home late quite often over the next few months. Harry promises to call. He also asks, "When I get home, please don't bombard me with problems. Let me have a few minutes to tune out the world. I need some real peace and quiet when I first get home. I feel so overloaded."

Martha responds empathically, "I can understand, dear, but I'm not sure it will be fair to the kids and me to see so little of you if you are consistently coming home late." Harry responds by promising to make the weekends a special time. Harry then tells her of some events at the office that caused him to feel quite worried that the promotion he has hoped for may go to someone who has less seniority. Both are able to pay attention to the words of the other and to make compromises. Both are willing to make an extra effort to solve the problem and ensure that it goes no further.

Now, consider the same situation when spouses are functioning at the intermediate level 2. Martha is angry because Harry is late; he forgot to call and dinner is ruined.

Martha says, "All you care about is work. You don't care about me. I've been standing over a hot stove after working hard all day. I need your help and support and so do the kids."

Harry responds, "All you ever do is nag. You don't care that I'm trying like hell to earn money to make life better for both of us."

"You are not trying to earn money for us. All you really want is to take care of yourself. You want to earn money so you can have a new Mercedes. You don't pay attention to me. I'm not important, your job is. What difference does it make if you earn more money if you're too tired when you come home to take time with your children, to go out to dinner with me, to have some fun, sometimes," says Martha in return.

To which Harry replies, "All you ever care about is having a good time. You don't care if I come home exhausted and tired and need a hot meal on the table."

"If you really want a hot meal, you've got one. Your dinner burned an hour ago and there is nothing else for you to eat." At this point, Harry decides to go to Joe's Bar to get a few stiff drinks. He comes home an hour later and looks in the refrigerator, knowing that she has left something for him to eat. "She may complain a lot," he thinks, "but she won't let me go hungry."

In this intermediate level 2 couple, there are occasional borderline defensive reactions. At that moment neither is able to recognize the separate needs or concerns of the other. Each blames and dumps out the anger toward the other. Anxiety, guilt, and neediness are passed back and forth between them, ultimately leading to retreat from the unresolvable situation. Each was upset and wished for understanding from the other. He withdrew; she was left with her anger. This occurs at sporadic times when one or both are under stress. Violent arguments alternate with days when they relate with a degree of comfort and affection.

Again, the same scenario but this time from the point of view of a couple at the more archaic level 1 border of pathological reactions: On the way home, Harry realizes that he forgot to call Martha. "Boy, am I in trouble. She is going to be mad. I guess I should have called, but she should understand that when the boss piles work on me I don't even have the time to stop and call. I don't know why I have to work so hard. I'm probably not going to get that promotion anyway. It's silly to have to work so hard and not come home until 8:30. If it weren't for her and the kids, I wouldn't have to work so hard. If she didn't spend so much, and got a job that paid more, I wouldn't have to work so hard. Why doesn't she stop complaining and nagging so much and make things easier for me. That's the way a woman should be, instead of always looking for something to fight about."

At this point, Harry is pulling into the driveway. Martha meets him at the door with her complaint that he should have called, because now his dinner is burned.

"You're just always looking for a fight, aren't you?" Harry screams. "I came home as soon as I could. What the hell do you know about working hard?"

Martha, used to these shouting matches, screams back, "You're no good. You're never here when I need you. The kids have been impossible, the house is dirty, and your dinner is a charred mess. You probably weren't working late at all and went out to a bar with those bums you call friends. You're just like my father, always out drinking with the guys. Get your own damn dinner. I'm not doing a thing for you."

Harry pushes her aside, angrily saying, "What a bitch. You should just be glad I'm home at all. It's my income that supports this house, and I can do anything I damn well please. Who needs you anyway?" He goes through the dining room and knocks a chair down to the floor, then slams the door as he walks out. He returns after midnight.

The next morning he comes down while Martha and the children are having breakfast. He speaks to her as though the argument the previous day had never happened. She is still angry and refuses to answer. They avoid talking for several days. One day they resume talking. As far as he is concerned, the argument is buried and never happened. Meanwhile, she is still boiling inside, but won't give him the satisfaction of telling him how hurt and upset she is. Martha feels agitated about her life most of the time, but her experience tells her that it is hopeless to try to change anything.

The examples above show how people at different levels along the narcissistic continuum deal with hurt, anger, and rage. The person who functions at the level of mature narcissism in relationships, although very upset, can contain the anger and maintain contact with both self and other.

The stressful experience does not cause fragmentation or loss of cohesion. The problem can be resolved in a manner that is not destructive to the relationship. In the latter scenario the couple operates in a narcissistic collusion using archaic defenses. For couples functioning at this level, the interaction centers around their deep primitive hurts and defenses. It begins with a fantasized discussion which takes on a reality of its own by the time Harry gets home. The interaction centers around such defenses as splitting and projective identification, the dumping of unacceptable aspects of the self into one another. Martha sees her angry unavailable father in Harry. She expects marriage to be a series of battles. In her husband she found the perfect fit for her expectations. Harry's anger was building up to explosive levels even before he walked in the door. Defending himself from his own inner dialogue, he quickly connected with a primitive level in his wife where her rageful reactions matched his. At that moment she feels only hate for him. She must keep her guard up at all times because he is so "crazy." Harry sees himself as the victim of her persecution.

He anticipates her responses because the script has been played out many times before. Their pathological interaction evokes behavior which, if described by either to a third party, would make the listener wonder how anyone could stand living with such a disturbed person.

Sometimes disturbed interactions make the persons involved function at a level that appears more pathological than is actually the case. Other times severe pathology is mitigated by a finely tuned positive relationship in which mates operate as good selfobjects for each other. Still other times a person may carry so heavy a burden of unresolved early experiences of emotional failures that unrealistic demands and defenses make relationships almost impossible. In the next section several different situations will be considered.

NARCISSISTIC DEFENSIVE ORGANIZATION IN RELATIONSHPS

Since people who fall in love and marry tend to have similar early developmental failures but opposite or complementary patterns of defensive organization (Gurman, 1978), the marital system may develop in ways that maintain the defensive patterns of each partner. The hurt, vulnerable self seeks opportunities for reparative experiences in relationships throughout life. Thus, there is a constant replay of the early injury.

Pathological interactions are characterized by repeated failure to recognize the feelings and needs of an intimate other or by an inability to experience another as anything more than a provider of gratification. Depending upon the type and depth of distortion, and the available internal resources, talents, and skills, narcissistic needs may be overtly acted out in grandiose fantasies and expectations, or covertly expressed by filling such needs in others. At times narcissistic conflicts lead to useful adaptations. For example, the need for empathic response and nurturance may be transformed into the capacity to understand the needs of others and may be played out in various roles, including that of psychotherapist.

Sometimes narcissistic pathology is mitigated by mutual support. Sally and Reggie are both psychotherapists. Both work with severely disturbed adolescents. Occasionally Reggie arranges for one of his patients to come home with him. He believes in total immersion in the treatment. Reggie freely admits that the craziness that he works with in his patients is a mirror image of what he sometimes sees in himself. He recalls hallucinating as an adolescent; even now, when he gets upset, he feels as though his mind is fragmenting. Sally knows her husband well. She knows that despite transient psychotic episodes, Reggie is a loving, caring man who does a great deal for his profession and his patients. She feels that he is not appreciated enough for all that he does, and she is always ready, like a lioness, to fight off anyone who threatens or hurts him. Occasionally he gets enraged or behaves inappropriately with her, but for the most part it is the two of them, against the world, joined together to fight off a common enemy. I doubt that Reggie would be a reasonably well-functioning person without Sally's support.

When partners feel safe enough to drop their shields with each other, they no longer need to put energy into defenses. Instead they have the freedom to explore themselves, to grow and test out changes. As that occurs they have more to share with each other and more energy to put into the relationship. They lose the fear that what will spontaneously emerge is dangerous, damaging, or destructive to themselves, others, or the relationship. Reggie's experience in the relationship has made him feel reassured that his words will not later come back as accusations or negative judgments. Criticism, while experienced at times as painful, is not viewed as intentionally designed to attack or hurt him, because it does not include an implication of abandonment or an accusation about something "bad" within.

Sometimes narcissistic needs are psychologically placed into another person under the erroneous assumption that what is given will be received with pleasure and reciprocated. Thus, we find the husband who thinks that by working very hard he is doing everything for his family, while neither his wife nor his children have a genuine relationship with him. Similarly, with righteous indignation a persons complains, "I am always helping others, but

I never get anything back." When one examines the transactions between narcissistically vulnerable mates, it often becomes apparent that what was given was neither requested nor wanted. The reenacted fantasy can take the form, "Because I love my partner, I know what (s)he thinks and wants."

At an unconscious level, the mate may be seen as a part of the self, an identical or Siamese twin; therefore, there is no need to articulate thoughts and desires. Boundaries are felt to be fluid and permeable, allowing either to get inside the other. Such open boundaries interfere with the ability to discriminate one's own thoughts, wishes, and intentions from the partner's and result in a sense of entitlement and confusion that covers a myriad of deep fears and self-hate. The complementary message is "Love means never having to say what I want; you should know. If I have to tell you what I want, even if you do it for me it doesn't count. If you loved me you would know without being told."

Where vulnerability is not extreme, there may still be temporary regressions to earlier developed narcissistic states. If the illusions of early narcissism are carried into adulthood, they interfere with the development of the necessary capacity to see an intimate other as having separate boundaries. The other is instead experienced as a continuation of the self, often carrying all the badness and craziness that cannot be borne within. Any suggestion of separateness or independence may occasion rage and even violence. Some narcissistically damaged adults expect to have the same kind of control over their mates and children as they do over parts of their own bodies (Kohut, 1977).

John and Audrey

John was a 32-year-old workaholic. At times he felt brilliant, successful, and omnipotent, but maintenance of this grandiosity was dependent on the responses of others around him at work and at home. He was particularly vulnerable to the opinions and reactions of his wife, Audrey. Her critical glances during the early years of their marriage punctured his inflated image of himself, leaving him empty and devastated. Audrey was 18 and very insecure when they met and married, all within a period of six weeks. Marriage to her was an opportunity to free herself from a rigidly controlling, fundamentalist religious family. She spent the first years of their marriage trying to decide "what I am going to be when I grow up." Art collecting had always interested her greatly, and she timorously began purchasing a few small pieces. Soon she decided to go to school to study art history. John subsidized her interest in art while intermittently letting her know that he thought her taste was abominable compared to his own well-trained eye for art. Her reaction to his belittling remarks was to spend more money on both paintings and clothing.

He used his money to meet her expensive tastes and to entertain her many artistic friends on the condition that he be included in all of her activities. At the same time as he damanded inclusion, he found fault constantly with the pretensions and talents of her friends.

When his wife's friends began to avoid him, he became indignant, pointing out all of the important people with whom he did business and who found his company quite acceptable. "They are all stupid and a waste of time to be with," he said, devaluating those who did not admire and accept him. He resented Audrey's wish to spend so much time with them.

Like many who are acting upon old narcissistic vulnerabilities, John was desperately looking for love and admiration. He surrounded himself with "friends" and attended many parties, always seeking more admiration and gratification. He considered himself sensitive to the needs of others and believed that he was constantly doing things for people who never reciprocated.

John never understood why people were so unappreciative. He failed to recognize that what he gave to others was actually what he wanted for himself and had little to do with what they might want. He had little true awareness of what his wife or friends wanted because he had limited awareness of them as separate people. It was a source of constant disappointment to him to be confronted with what he experienced as unreasonable demands by others.

John's history reveals a legacy of an unhappy home, in which neither parent spent very much time with their children. He was raised by a series of housekeepers and babysitters, and recalls fighting with them all. Throughout his early life he experienced clashing interactions with others. There was repeated confirmation that what he must do in his current relationships was exactly what he had been doing throughout his life. It felt right, yet it seemed to result in constant anguish.

His way of life was a continuation of an earlier need for "merger" as a young child with a depressed mother. His mother was unresponsive emotionally unless he generated enough energy and excitement to capture her interest and attention. He made himself a source of aliveness for her, no matter how he felt himself. He learned early that the ways that most people find comfort, reassurance, and human contact as a separate, autonomous human being could not work for him. In his current relationships he lives psychologically in the past. If one appreciates the interpersonal consequences of having lived life this way for many years, John's idiosyncratic version of reality does not seem quite so out of tune with his world.

While John's way of viewing his relationships was more distorted than most, everyone lives in a world infused with his or her particular personality. Each of us actually does encounter different events and receive different responses from those experienced by others (Wachtel and Wachtel, 1986). How we select relationships and respond in interactions causes others to react in certain anticipated ways. Each person, thus, creates a "subjective," idiosyncratic way of experiencing situations.

John, expecting to be hurt and needing to control, selected for a mate Audrey, whose history was one of struggling for separateness and independence. She found this struggle recreated in her marriage. Progressively each moved to more extreme versions of their characteristic ways of functioning. John did not relate to his wife as an autonomous person, instead treating her as an extension of himself. She said that she felt like one of his possessions. "He has his boat, his Mercedes, his tennis court, and his wife." She did not feel she could have needs of her own, but must exist solely to take care of him, to be an adjunct to his existence, making him feel whole and complete.

Beneath John's demands and blustering rages is an extraordinary fear that separation will cause painful loss and abandonment. Audrey knows that his financial support of her art and her way of life will keep her tied to him, but she distances herself from him in many ways. She experiences his needs as demanding that she sacrifice herself, living completely and only for him. She does not get her own needs met and has put up a defensive wall to protect herself against his intrusions. Increasingly, she has turned to her friends for affirmation. Neither knows how to change the script. Each chooses to accept the unfulfilling relationship rather than risk its complete loss by attempting a change. The unknown dread is more terrifying than known discontent.

The relationship between John and Audrey is an extreme example of an oppositional merger-separation struggle into an adult relationship. It is one of many such conflicts in which the early narcissistic injury of each mate turns into a marital collusion in which each seeks in the other a reparative experience; then, when the relationship fails to meet expectations, it turns into a pattern of attack and defense operations.

A CASE OF SEVERE PERSONALITY DISORDER

While most people are subject to regressions when they undergo high stress or narcissistic injury, some function at this lower level as a general condition. Early injury for such people has kept them in a phase of primitive affective reactions and archaic defense mechanisms. At times the pathology is so severe that mutually enhancing relationships are not possible. Twenty-five-year-old Bart has a severe personality disorder in which he experiences his internal world as chaotic, terrifying, full of uncontrollable rage. A budding rock musician with orange speckled hair and two earrings in his right ear, he said he always knew that he was defective. In therapy he reported stories he had heard of being so awful as a child that, after his father brought him home from the adoption agency, his mother locked the door and hid from him. He tried, he said, to be normal all of his life, but could not seem to do it. Even while he sat and talked, Bart's body was in constant motion. He had always been hyperactive—no asset in a home where the mother objected to having a second child and agreed to the adoption only under the threat of divorce. The father desperately wanted to have a son and used his power and financial position to adopt when his wife was unable to conceive. But the father did not have the capacity to overcome the mother's apparent inability to bond or respond. Bart's explanation of what was wrong was that he was defective—and that is what made his mother not want to touch him. "I was expelled from two nursery schools—I must have been pretty awful," he repeated several times. He never did adjust to a school setting or a job. He did have some talent in music and found a place for himself where he was almost accepted, but always felt on the periphery. Any close relationship terrified him, yet he said that he wished he could find someone to love him. His severe borderline pathology has made him almost nonfunctioning.

THE NEED FOR AFFIRMATION

Narcissism, then, is not simply self-centeredness, nor is it always a symptom of severe pathology. There is a wide variation in the narcissistic continuum, from the personalized idiosyncratic world view of mature narcissistic levels to the almost nonfunctional archaic levels of primitive terror and defense. It can range from an extraordinary sensitivity to the moods and feelings of important others, which is the basis of empathy, to an exquisite sense of emotional injury at the slightest failures of needed response. This sensitivity to psychic damage develops during the earliest life interactions and is recreated in certain later situations.

No matter how limited the person or how severe the disorder, there is a basic human need to be recognized for who one is to be accepted, affirmed, and secure in the feeling of being part of a loving relationship.

Failure to meet the needs for affirming, caring, emotional connections anywhere in the life cycle is likely to cause psychological, relational, and/or physical symptoms. Unresponsiveness to needs in early development put the child at risk for future narcissistic vulnerability. Chapter 4 will review developmental factors and early interactions influencing the world view of each person. We will see how the primary interactions are the building blocks of a lifetime of relationships, and become the basis of both health and pathology.

The Origins of Narcissistic Disorders

To some extent the perceptions of all of us are colored and distorted. Experiences in infancy and early childhood accumulate as a prototype, a personal world view that affects all interpersonal relations. "All human relationships are experienced through a lens formed of a multitude of other experiences, remembered or not" (Will, 1987, p. 257). Depending upon the lens through which we have learned to look, each new relationship will be entered into with some combination of trust, hope, and fear.

Our recollection of events is based upon how they were first experienced and how later experiences transformed the earlier memories. Subjective memories of events develop layer upon layer and become the building blocks of interactions that are later recalled in interpersonal relationships. Some disturbances in early life events distort perceptions of self and other. Defensive measures, strategies devised to protect a vulnerable self from overwhelming distress, are needed by the infant experiencing an emotionally or physically precarious situation. Later these defenses may be reintroduced when interpersonal experiences include a spark reminiscent of archaic fears. Every person develops an elaborate system of beliefs, thoughts, and expectations of self and other that may be referred to as a "personal theory of reality" (Epstein, 1973, p. 404)—a personal world view.

A personal theory of reality assimilates and "formats" an individual's experiences, maintains self-esteem, and creates a stable balance over the foreseeable future. It includes concepts of what is internal "me" and external "not me," self and other, as well as the capacity for personal meaning and value. Looking through the filter of a personal world view, each individual in a different way experiences emotion and sensuality, beauty and ugliness, hopes for the future, memories of the past, lushness or emptiness of internal life.

The result is a "working model" of self-other interactions that is maintained with little variation during the course of a lifetime. Messages sent consciously and unconsciously encourage reciprocal reactions from others that confirm the previously developed internal model. Interpersonal history is, thus, preordained to repeat itself unless new, modifying forces are introduced. The flexibility and responsiveness to new learning of this pattern of interactions is one important measure of mental health. The more the pattern is fixed, the greater is the restriction in range of responses.

Although we know that experiences are incorporated from the beginning of life, infant researchers differ on what the earliest interpersonal experiences are. Although Mahler identifies an early symbiotic phase, others suggest that from the first weeks, the infant is aware of and responds to the world outside itself. This will be discussed later. Based upon the fit of needs and caretaking responses, expectations develop about future interactions. This generates patterns of behavior that elicit confirmation of a set of expectations and self-fulfilling prophecies about ways of being in the world.

CHRISTIE'S FIGHT FOR A SELF OF HER OWN

Many well-meaning parents are determined to do everything for their child. They project onto their offspring all of the idealized perfection that they wish for themselves: "The baby will have all of the love that I was lacking as a baby. This child will never be left in the care of babysitters, or housekeepers, as I always was. . . . I will make sure that my baby will not be afraid, confused, hurt, needy. . . . This child will get the chance that I never had." A child who is programmed to live out the parents' dreams may rebel in any number of ways, whether as a "terrible two" or as a rebellious adolescent. Such parents are generally frustrated and disappointed when their child fights for a singular personality.

Christie's parents, Richard and Margaret, both had very strong needs for acceptance and emotional security in a relationship. Their marriage was a merger. They had great expectations for relationships, and they met many of these expectations for each other. They are both painters. When I met them 11 years ago, they were both unknown, but over the years Richard has become quite famous for his work. Margaret never had any serious conflicts about choosing between pursuing a career and being a wife and mother. While she occasionally paints, marriage and children have always been her top priority. As both are over six feet tall, they are a striking couple and they know it. Whatever their goals, they expect to do them well. When I first met them, they had just celebrated their ninth wedding anniversary. They did not request marital therapy, but consultation about their child, before she was born.

For their first eight years of marriage they had been unable to have a child because of a physical problem Margaret had. Both desperately wanted children and put a great deal of their emotional energy into obsessing over their unfulfilled desire for children. During the early years of their marriage each babied the other. They traveled together, supported each other in highly creative careers, and advised friends on how to be happily married and how to raise children.

After eight years of trying, Margaret became pregnant. They rearranged their home and their lifestyle with the intention of bringing up a perfectly behaved, highly successful child who would bring joy to their lives. They sought therapeutic consultation as a kind of prebirthing counseling. Was there anything that they might have missed, they asked, that would add to their joint fantasy of producing the perfect baby? While they appeared to ask questions, in fact they had all the answers.

They were clearly not interested in any cautions about placing unrealistic expectations on their child. They knew exactly what was wrong with the way all of their friends raised children. Their child would never be left with a babysitter other than one of the grandparents. Nor would he or she be spoiled, overfed with sweets, or allowed indiscriminate television watching. In fact, they intended to be perfect parents and demonstrate to their friends, whose children were all spoiled, how to raise a child.

When their baby girl, Christie, was born they sent me a card, and I wrote back asking them to keep in touch to let me know how their childrearing plans were progressing. Every December I got a newsletter full of the year's family happenings. From their reports, they had followed through on their plans to never leave their daughter without one of them or a grandparent in attendance. Their daughter seemed to be progressing remarkably well. She was precocious, gifted musically, and an outstanding student. Her mother gave up her career and became a housewife, girl scout leader, and editor of the school newsletter. The parents went on vacations with her and took her whenever they were invited to friends' homes. If friends disapproved, they gave up the friends.

Occasionally the parents came in to talk about a particular issue concerning Christie. At times I observed Margaret's almost manic behavior. When I commented on it, she said at first that it was due to some diet pills that she was taking. However, by the time Christie was ten it was clear that her mother was dealing with her problems by overusing amphetamines and drinking too much. Christie was not turning out at all as she expected, nor was the marriage going well.

Christie herself complained that there was no "Christie" in this family. She was not allowed privacy or the freedom to have her own ideas. Her parents expected her to include them in all of her activities and wanted her to be part of whatever they did. As Christie had increasingly challenged her mother's values and ideas, Margaret felt hurt and angry. She began to feel that Christie and Richard were joining together and leaving her out.

Margaret had turned to substance abuse to relieve her increasing inner fears and turmoil. As long as Richard saw the problem between them as due to Margaret's drinking and amphetamine use, he and Christie could join together and condemn mother, thereby bringing the couple closer to divorce. Not until the family accepted the fact that this was a problem shared by all and recognized the need for help could anything change. Fortunately, they undertook therapy as thoroughly as they did everything else. A combination of AA meetings, individual and family therapy helped them to redirect the collusive, damaging pattern that was causing each of them a great deal of emotional pain. In individual therapy Christie began working to repair and strengthen some of the damaged self structures resulting from being raised by parents who "cared too much" and knew her too little.

EARLY DEVELOPMENTAL FACTORS

Current developmental research provides important clues not only to how infants learn to generalize experiences that become their unique representational models of the world, but also to how adults draw upon affective and emotional responses learned before verbal skills emerge in the attempt to communicate needs and experiences. When early development is proceeding normally, "there are likely to be flickering moments of awareness of bodily separateness from the mother even from the very beginning of life" (Tustin, 1987, p. 43). The infant has a preadaptive readiness to relate and to contribute to interactions with the environment, as well as a capacity to involve the caretaker in the kind of dialogue and interactions necessary for a mutuality of attachment. Nevertheless, individual constitutional differences in ability to regulate arousal and tolerance for stimulation may affect the infant's capacity to respond to caretakers and to tolerate environmental stresses (Stern, 1985). For example, certain genetic predispositions may precipitate the experience of emotional impoverishment in early nurturing. In most cases, when the primary and legitimate desire for emotional expression and genuine sensation is met, the self develops with a feeling of cohesiveness and durability. Figure 4.1 outlines the sequence of development of the self.

The first reactions of the infant are adaptive to the environmental factors experienced. These adaptations may later be found in distorted form as defensive measures that were appropriate responses at earlier times but are no longer fitting in current situations. Pathology is the continuation of prior adaptive measures as though the earlier interactional situation was manifesting itself in the present.

AN ILLUSION OF ONENESS

As the first diagram in Figure 4.1 suggests, the first two months mark a time in which "the infant is not related in any distinctive or unique way to other persons. Interpersonal relatedness does not yet exist as distinct from relatedness to things" (Stern, 1985, p. 63). Some see this time of development as a phase of undifferentiation, during which the infant subjectively experiences fusion or moments of merger (Pine, 1986a). Infants are, in actuality, active participants in an adaptive interaction with their environment from the time of birth onward, but subjectively they have little awareness of a world external to themselves.

Many well-functioning adults appear to carry an illusion of oneness, a memory of a sense of well-being in union with another, and a powerful wish to return to this benevolent state. Romantic love, the early period in an intimate relationship, appears as a re-creation of this experience. Marked by a joyful coming together, a desire to avoid any separation, a wish to share in everything with the other, it is reminiscent of a totally fused state of existence. A deep pain arises from physical, emotional, or sexual separation.

At some point in the developmental process recognition of the separateness of self and other begins. During this process an awareness of the existence of the other is transient and the boundaries between self and other are highly permeable. Winnicott (1971) describes the way the mother and child interact during this period as a holding zone—a transitional state. With this holding environment as a base the child moves into an awareness of others as separate beings. Through many ongoing interactions the "good enough mother" described by Winnicott expresses a capacity to emotionally hold the child and contain anxiety to a tolerable level, enabling the child to organize his or her own self.

While recognizing the reality of other's existence, there is a deeply felt inner state of need and sometimes an uncomfortable awareness of depen-

EMERGENT SELF
(Birth to two months)

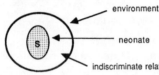

environment

neonate

indiscriminate relatedness to things/objects

CORE SELF
(two to six months)

infant   caretaker

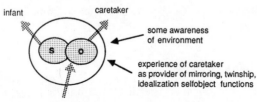

some awareness
of environment

experience of caretaker
as provider of mirroring, twinship,
idealization selfobject functions

intersubjective
experience of
self and object

Working model of mother
begins in infant's mind.

Authorship of actions.
Boundaries.
Sense of enduring self.
Encoding, integrating,
generalizing
guide behavior.
Core relatedness.
More integrated sense of self
as separate and distinct
from others.

SUBJECTIVE SELF
(seven to twelve months)

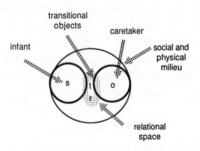

transitional
objects
caretaker

infant   social and
physical
milieu

relational
space

Use of transitional objects
between inner world and
environmental world.
Intersubjective relatedness
built on core of emergent self.
Sense of physical separateness.
Potential for sharing
subjective experience
and affective states.
Affect attunement.
Potential for empathy.
Need for inclusion in human group.

VERBAL SELF
(Second year of Life)

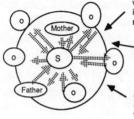

various levels of
interaction with
many others

potential for
verbal communication
and empathy

ability to hide
affect and feeling
with words

Sense of a verbal self
Ability to determine what to
communicate and what
remains private

Some loss of direct contact
with internal experience
due to lack of sufficient words
to identify the wide range of
affect and emotion in any
human being

FIGURE 4.1

dence on another. The danger in this period occurs when the primary caretaker, who is still experienced as a needed extension of the self, is temporarily damaged or chronically not present to meet the infant's needs. The grief and detachment that ensue can permeate all later relationships. This may be denied through a merger fantasy. The conflict later can manifest as a need to fuse with an idealized other who can read one's mind and respond immediately in a perfect caretaking function, as in the marriage of John and Audrey described in Chapter 3.

THE SELF IN CONTEXT

We cannot speak of an individual without recognizing that the self exists only in context. Anna and Paul Ornstein (1985) note that the self can be conceptualized as an "experiential unit," self and other in reciprocal relationship. On a similar note, Winnicott (1958) said there is no such thing as an infant, but only an infant-mother dyad. In infancy, there is a basic drive toward an integrated self existing along with relatedness to others. When early development fails to provide the necessary and sufficient conditions for consolidation of a cohesive self and trust in the integrity of self-other boundaries, interpersonal relatedness is affected. Whether others are experienced as whole individuals or simply as objects designed to meet personal needs depends crucially on these early developmental interchanges. The particulars of early experience are replayed in later intimate attachments.

We do not know with any certainty why some individuals emerge from infancy more damaged than others and carry that damage with them the rest of their lives. Kohut (1971) noted that the complexity of the interplay between parent and child defies comprehensive description. We are only beginning to develop a systematic understanding of the causes of psychological problems and of the internal experience of the infant. However, we can say with some assurance that many of the presenting problems seen in psychotherapists' offices stem from a combination of genetic predisposition and interaction with the environment during the early years of life (Bowlby, 1969; Mahler, et al., 1975; Winnicott, 1965). The brain, the mind, the body, the family, and society all contribute to development of a personal world view, which in turn affects interpersonal relatedness. The interaction of these factors from the beginning of life helps to structure the developing sense of self.

THE DEVELOPMENT OF A SENSE OF SELF

Varying senses of self develop, not as phases that are outgrown but as aspects of the personality that remain and reemerge at various points in life

(Stern, 1985). Nothing is lost; rather, each state is reexperienced as events later in life trigger certain memories. "The advent of a higher stage does not destroy the earlier phase, rather it embraces its own perspective" (Cassiver, 1955, p. 477). Mahler also recognized that developmental "phases" are not time-limited. She saw each phase as reverberating "throughout the life cycle. It is never finished; it remains always active; new phases of the life cycle see new derivatives of the earliest process still at work" (Mahler et al., 1975, p. 3). Every subsequent interaction is built upon a past history of intersubjective experiences between child and caretaker.

Figure 4.2 describes several levels of relatedness in the early developmental sequences between the developing child and caretaker. In the first weeks of life the infant's experiences include some recognition of the sight, smell and sound of mother's presence; relatedness is emerging (Stern, 1985).

Beginning as early as two months of age there is a building of interactional events that result in a core relatedness, a recognition of self and otherness. By seven months, the infant is already involved in a series of differing interactions that may include peaceful merger (Pine, 1986a), alert activity, or moments of anxiety. It is a period of intersubjective relatedness. As the child learns to talk, there is a beginning of verbal relatedness and a new ability to determine what will be publicly shared and what remains in the private domain of the self. At the same time there is some loss of contact with direct experience, affectivity for which words are not available (Stern, 1985).

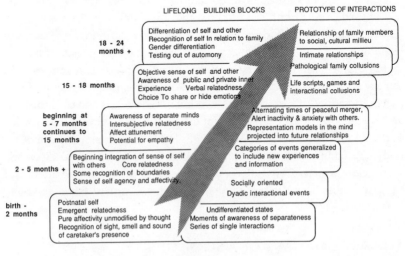

FIGURE 4.2

Developmental Sequences in Early Life:
Building Blocks of a Lifetime of Relationships

By the 18th month there is a differentiation of self and other, an awareness of gender, anxieties related to bodily cohesion, and development of autonomous functions. The child comes to differentiate the boundaries of self and other, often expressing verbally the autonomy of the self. The period that follows is generally known as the "terrible twos," in which the word "no" is commonly used to express separateness and individuation. At this point also there is the awareness of gender differentiation along with oedipal fantasies. Oedipal issues have been examined by many of the classical analysts, beginning with Freud. While they are an important aspect of the relationships between children and parents, and between husband and wife, they will not be detailed here, since our focus is on the narcissistic aspects that precede the oedipal phase.

The most significant issues in determination of adult relationships are the earliest interactions, the emergent and core relatedness patterns seen in Figure 4.2. At this time of life the issues focus on the need for and maintenance of contacts with others. At the archaic and intermediate transitional levels (see Figure 3.1) the primary anxieties center around survival, identity, and existence. Borderline and psychotic defenses that develop at this time have their derivation in pre-oedipal phases.

The work done by Freud and the classical analysts was concerned with the genitality, repressed sexuality, and oedipal feelings, sexual and competitive, of the child who has mastered the earlier developmental stages. At the level of object constancy the mother is perceived and recalled even in her temporary absence. The baby has learned to trust that, although she is gone at the moment, she will reemerge soon enough. However, prior to the achievement of awareness that other human beings exist even when they are not immediately present, and prior to a recognition that there are two sexes, each with different physiologies, there is already a world filled with interactional events that are generalized perceptions of relatedness. In this world narcissistic vulnerability has its origins.

Investigators such as Fairbairn (1954a), Kohut (1977), and Greenberg and Mitchell (1983) have noted the frequency with which sexual conflicts and wishes are the vehicle for other, often earlier, infantile thoughts and impulses involving dependency longings. Fairbairn indicated that libido is not pleasure-seeking but object-seeking, and that pleasure is not the end goal of an impulse but a means to an end — relations with another. Genitality, then, is not the major basis for adult intimacy but rather one channel for its expression.

How the developing child reacts to awareness of genitality has already been determined by internalized representations of mother, father, and self. These are based upon internal representational models that become prototypes for all future experiences. The additional experiences during the oedipal period will then be projected onto future relationships. It is the development of these earliest relationships, generalized and incorporated into prototypical interactions, which strongly affects the patterns that are later seen in marital and family therapy.

There is a critical period during which maintaining social contact and forming attachments are both necessary for survival, even when frustrating. In this process healthy defenses are essential to the formation of psychic structure. In an idealized developmental sequence, the newborn infant encounters a perfect environment, a nurturing, responsive relationship totally attuned and available to precisely reflect and meet the baby's needs as experienced. In this way the infant becomes attuned to his/her own bodily functions and impulses. These become the basis for a growing, slowly evolving sense of self. "When I look I am seen, so I exist" (Winnicott, 1971, p. 134). If only this idealized set of events occurred, however, it would make learning difficult. What makes learning possible is the mother's occasional failure to shape the world according to the baby's needs and demands (Kohut, 1971; Winnicott, 1958).

In normal development there are many small failures—no parent is perfectly attuned and available to respond ideally at all times. The "good enough" mother's failures enable the child to develop tolerance of frustration, recognition of others, and internal self structures. The child who learns that gratification does not come immediately but occurs within a reasonable period of time comes to terms with inner needs and outer providers and can perceive the environment as benign and caring.

RECIPROCITY OF MOTHER, FATHER, AND CHILD

We cannot assess the state of the developing child's sense of self without considering the way in which the emerging self is experiencing and internalizing its emotional environment. Nor can we make an assessment of parental responsiveness without understanding the impact of the developing, changing child on the mother and father at any particular point in time. A child who, for whatever reason, encounters difficulty in the course of development will affect the parents' self-esteem to various degrees. It is the parents' narcissistic investment in the child that assures adequate care (Ornstein and Ornstein, 1985). With each child, at each new stage of development, the parents' empathic capacities are tested anew.

Even before an infant is born, the parents place many expectations, hopes, and problems onto the baby-to-be in an idealized fantasy of hope that this continuation of themselves will provide for their own unconscious needs. Many projections are passed from grandparents to parents and on to the next generation without any conscious awareness of the process. The mother's unconscious is the child's first reality (McDougall, in press). "The human infant is exposed to the anxieties, beliefs, values, emotions, ways of living, and personal idiosyncrasies of those who care for him. During his early life he is bound to a narrow space, physically and socially, from which he cannot escape" (Will, 1980, p. 1230). A caretaker's insecurity, whatever its source, can lead to a number of unfortunate consequences. Normal imperfections in the developing child may be viewed as defects, fatal flaws that interfere with a parent's fantasy of a perfect child. The child may be needed to mobilize the unresolved issues and narcissistic vulnerabilities in the parents.

At later points in development the child's normal search for separateness and autonomy may be experienced as threatening by a parent who needs the symbiotic closeness of no boundaries. This child may then suppress independent wishes and needs in an effort to assure continuing love and protection (Masterson, 1981). Since the kind of responsiveness expressed in the nurturing role is parallel to the caretaker's own early experiences with significant others, patterns are perpetuated from generation to generation.

Just as behaviors of mother and child influence each other, the father's relationships with both mother and child have a tremendous influence on development of the emerging self of the child. A new pregnancy, for example, is assimilated into a woman's sense of herself. The reaction of her husband to her pregnancy and motherhood can have a profound impact on her experience (Atwood and Stolorow, 1984). A mother who has a precarious sense of self or who does not feel content with the emotional supplies provided by her husband may come to rely on her baby to fulfill her own archaic needs for connection with others.

The responses of the infant to mother and father also contribute to the intersubjective field that arises between parent and child. Since caretakers respond selectively to a few of many varied cues presented by the infant, behavior is gradually shaped in specific directions. A pattern of interaction that constitutes the child's personality emerges from the combination of innate endowment and the parent-child relationship. Early interactions, therefore, create the "child" out of the infant's infinite potentialities (Stern, 1985). In like manner, each child "creates'" his own mother and father as the parents' empathic responses dovetail with the specific needs of the particular child (Ornstein and Ornstein, 1985).

For example, a quiet and passive child for whom "good enough" mothering would mean a peaceful and nonstimulating environment might be overwhelmed by an active, stimulating, fast-paced mother (Escalona, 1968), while a child who can tolerate the rapid pace might benefit from interaction with such a mother. On the other hand, a child who is quiet and with-drawn might benefit from a high level of stimulation and atrophy emotion-ally if cared for by a quiet parent. The match of child to parent has a lot to do with memories the child carries into later life, as well as with the child's attempts to make up in some way for what is missing. Disease is never merely a loss or excess; there is always a reaction on the part of the affected organism or individual—to restore, to replace, to compensate, to preserve and restore identity, however strange the means may appear to be (Sacks, 1985).

Some children who are particularly attuned and sensitive to the needs of others may become "parentified," assuming the role of emotional caretaker for the parents (Miller, 1981). This may occur as a result of the parent's circumstantial or characterological needs. The mother may be depressed, alcoholic, emotionally withdrawn, or physically ill. The child is subtly induced to become the provider of nurturance or affirmation. Aspects of the self deemed unacceptable, those filled with the child's needs, intense emotions, or thoughts, may have to be denied or left underdeveloped in exchange for being loved by the parents. While appearing mature at an early age, and presenting a strong outward appearance, such children hold in feelings of longing and rage (McDougall, in press).

Palombo's (1987) research into the early lives of so-called "borderline" patients and P. Kernberg's (1984) discussion of the assessment of children with "borderline" personality organization confirm that psychological and subsequent relationship problems are multiply caused. In particular, the presence of neuropsychological problems in borderline children can lead to hyperactivity, learning disabilities and difficulties in social interaction; these compound their psychological problems and add to their inability to cope.

Some young infants are excessively sensitive to stimulation. "Noise in the psychic system" interferes with the ability to form, integrate, and maintain certain early critical developmental achievements (Pine, 1986b) and may encourage withdrawal into a narcissistic shell that will protect the vulnera-ble child from a barrage of stimuli (Grotstein, 1987). Such a situation hampers the possibility of receiving optimal mothering. Oversensitivity to stimulation is an instance of a neurological factor that predisposes the child to emotional disturbance.

Carl, for example, was always sensitive to noise and movement, reacting constantly to the activities taking place in his home. His memory of a busy environment was confirmed in a family-of-origin session (Framo, 1982). The household included parents, grandparents, and a series of immigrant relatives who lived there temporarily. Carl's parents, however, did not consider the household particularly noisy, nor did they understand the shell that he constructed about himself. Carl felt different from his cousins and friends and always wondered why.

Carl reported in therapy that he spent his entire childhood trying to fit in. For years he thought that in time he would feel "normal." As an adult, he is professionally successful but continues to have great difficulty sustaining and tolerating close interactions. He goes to parties, he says, but then he retreats to a quiet room. Sometimes he sits in the dark and listens to the others laugh and enjoy themselves. He wishes to be with others but to remain in the background. The world of others seems an intrusion from which he has to shield himself. Other people seem "like sandpaper," always rubbing him the wrong way.

The child's experience determines whether a stimulus or event is traumatic: "It is not the objective behavior of the other, but rather how that behavior is experienced . . . that is laid down in memory and carried . . . and how the other is experienced depends upon the child's affective, cognitive, and need state of the moment" (Pine, 1986b, p. 452). In Carl's case, his relatively low threshold for excitation, not parental abuse or neglect, forced him into the narcissistic position of demanding interaction with others on his own idiosyncratic terms.

THE DESIRE FOR AND AVOIDANCE OF RELATIONSHIPS

Carl sought therapeutic help when he recognized that he did not want to spend his entire life alone, and yet did not know how to love anyone. When he was alone he thought that he should be with people but when he was with others he felt estranged and disconnected. Any attempt by others to reach out to Carl, any offer of human contact, was responded to by distancing and retreat. In his work he fended off boredom and restlessness through research and writing that gained for him national prominence in his field. Outside of work he filled himself with classical music and the purchase of art. "I feel like a color-blind man who hears descriptions of beautiful colors, but can see only in black and white. I want more, so much more," he said with a sadness and hopelessness that I could feel to my depths.

Barry too, wished for and feared a relationship. At the age of 40 he decided that he was getting older and would like to marry and have a family. At that point he realized that he did not know how to feel close to a woman, although he had dated many. Thinking back during a therapy session, he remembered how often women had complained about his uncommitted non-involvement in relationships. As he recalled his past, he was reminded of his mother, whom everyone considered ideal. Barry remembered only a mother who was always out "doing good" for some cause. He could not recall being held, talked to, or asked about his interests. Barry recalled consciously deciding never to expect anything from his mother and never to share anything that was within him. He withheld from her any opportunity to enjoy his success. When she was dying he thought of telling her that he loved her, but he could not. He had not learned how to experience or verbalize feelings.

His early painful lack of an empathic or mirroring response followed him throughout his adult life. It made him fearful of lowering the wall of defenses that had protected him from emotional injury and, therefore, from emotional contact or love. Although neither Barry nor his father was physically demonstrative, he knew that his father cared a great deal about him. As a child, Barry knew that, if he mentioned to his father that he needed or wished for some particular toy or dessert or equipment for school, his father would not forget. Barry's feeling that he was valuable to his father, as well as the knowledge that there was someone he could trust, made it possible for him to begin repairing the damage he sustained in his internal experience of a nonempathic relationship with his mother.

THE BASIS OF LIFELONG RELATIONSHIPS

The actual experiences of Carl in his environment and the relationship between Barry, his mother, and his father can only be assumed. Much of what is described in the psychiatric literature about early development is based upon reports by adults in treatment. The recreation of the early relationship in the transference provides some insight into the past, and we are currently learning a great deal about development by direct observation of infants. Mahler and her associates (1975) observed young babies and came to some important new understanding of developmental phases. However, some of the conclusions in their book *The psychological birth of the human infant: Symbiosis and individuation* (1975) have been challenged by more recent research. Mahler describes an early undifferentiated symbiotic state followed by increasingly mature phases of separation and individuation. As we have seen, current research in infant development indicates that, rather than being unable to recognize the existence of a world outside the self, infants take in a wealth of information and respond to the environment through various sensory modalities (Stern, 1985).

We can see, then, how a number of factors, including temperament and responsiveness on the part of child and parents, influences the way each individual develops the resources necessary to meet the vicissitudes of life.

The fit between parent and child has important implications for what each gives and receives emotionally in the relationship. The coping mechanisms for psychic survival constructed during the early years—the inadequate, distorting adaptations of childhood—may later become the target of psychotherapeutic treatment.

In Dicks' early work on treatment of marital dysfunctions (1967) he observed that marriage is the nearest adult equivalent of the infant's bond with the primary caretaker. For those who have some capability to enter into intimate relationships, the process of falling in love recreates a fantasy of blissful merger of two selves. It is probable that at an unconscious level mate selection is a wish to return to the pleasures, the safety, the comfort of dependency, or to reenact what was missing in order to find a corrective emotional response reparative of early damaged relationships.

What occurs in the process of falling in love is a spark of recognition, a glimmer of memory of long-lost emotions. There is an unconscious wish for a reexperience of caregiving and hope for an experience that will repair what was lacking. Because this dynamic goes on without conscious awareness over a long period of time, old patterns may be endlessly replayed without successfully changing anything.

The narcissistic dilemma lies in the paradox of intimacy. Immersion into an intimate relationship means allowing one's sense of self to be merged or fused with another. This presents a danger. There is a fear of losing one's sense of self altogether. By using others as selfobjects, thus denying their separateness, one maintains an illusion of safety. Even if the adult is aware of this wish, the use of another to provide the selfobject functions, i.e., merger, soothing, affirming or twinship, is part of the private world of inner experience (see Figure 4.1). It is not something we talk about with our lovers. But this archaic wish is often acted upon in intimate relationship.

Many times the responses most wished for are those directed toward the most infantile, dependent aspects of the self. "Love all of me" is the message, although seldom is one able to admit this, since that would lead to too great a vulnerability. "Understand what I need" is the silent plea. "Make a place for my emotions, especially the ones that I cannot tolerate in myself."

It means intermittently allowing times of weakness and dependency, an emotional comfort zone, an island of safety secured by love and acceptance. It includes, in some instances of severe pathology, a recognition by the mate of occasional bizarre or crazy thoughts and a belief that such recognition will not cause the partner to withdraw in horror. Such an emotional comfort zone may occur anywhere throughout the course of life, from infancy onward. Ideally, it takes place first in the earliest relationships where the core self begins to emerge in relationship to others. If it does not, the emergence of a cohesive and enduring self may occur in intimate relationship later in life, but it will be more problematical.

In many relationships, and certainly in most that arrive in therapists' offices, the partners are not able to recognize or acknowledge each other's immature or archaic needs. There must be a willingness to listen to more than the surface level and to empathically acknowledge the internal experience of the other. Empathy requires not action, but understanding of core needs, affects, emotions and feelings. It is in this process that conjoint marital therapy can be useful.

As we have seen, narcissism occurs on a continuum and is not simply a pathology that interferes with intimacy. Some degree of narcissistic orientation permeates most intimate relationships. The narcissistic continuum is activated by various combinations of early interactional experiences and the dilemma of living in a narcissistic society. Depending upon the degree of narcissistic vulnerability, powerful emotional injury leading to shame or humiliation or massive disappointment in the archaic wish for a perfect love may cause a range of defenses to emerge. How these defenses operate to protect a vulnerable person is the subject of the next chapter.

CHAPTER 5

The Affect-Emotion-Feeling Triad

Each phase of development throughout life provides new challenges and dangers. This chapter discusses various affective, emotional, and feeling experiences, considers at which developmental level they emerge, and looks at the defenses that are used to ward off those experiences that threaten self-cohesion. It is important to understand the differences among affect, emotion and feeling in the internal experience, because the adult, in highly stressful or anxiety-provoking situations, is likely to regress to one of these earlier ways of reacting.

Affect, emotion, and feeling, each stemming alone or in combination from normal responses learned during successive developmental phases, surface pathologically when the raw nerve of the early developmental experiences is touched by the events of adult life. This discussion will include a theory which discriminates among and defines the affective, emotional, and feeling processes and describes their relation to the marital system.

Many deep internal experiences remain out of the conscious sphere because they developed before cognitive capacities evolved. There is no direct access to the affective experiences of the most archaic level, as they originated prior to development of words to identify them. Some painfully intense affect remains throughout life. Although it is not part of conscious awareness, it is often behaviorally or psychosomatically acted out.

Defenses develop to protect the self from unacceptable emotional pain. When feelings are powerful and the situation is experienced as dangerous, defenses are called into play to preserve self-cohesion. The early relationship with parents largely determines the nature and form of the defensive structures maintained throughout life. The greater the intimacy with another person, the more likely that early emotions and their defenses, perhaps along with archaic affects, will reemerge.

When resistances and defenses create problems in living, people may attempt to understand themselves better by entering psychotherapy. There they carefully associate words to unknown senses, peeling away and allowing into conscious awareness hidden layers of feelings, as well as emotions and affect. For many the goal is to discover the hidden core that has created disorders of life-functioning. Therapists develop skills for listening to the archaic messages, the interactionally generated emotions and the thought-out feelings beneath the resistances and defenses. They learn to listen empathically and to interpret what has been cut off and long-hidden from awareness. The psychotherapist's office is one place where early interactional experiences and defenses reemerge. Marriage is another.

Husbands and wives are not each other's therapists. They do not consistently attempt to listen attentively to one another's deepest fears and fantasies. Nor are they generally eager to provide security for the archaic core selves of one another. When hurt or upset themselves, they say and do things that can be damaging to the partner. Such statements as, "Why can't you ever get anything right?" "Get out of this house," and "I hate you," are part of the everyday discourse of many couples. These apparently hostile attacks may actually be a self-protective strategy used when there is a perceived injury or unfulfilled need in the relationship. What is being defended against is often unknown to either mate. It may lie deep within the archaic layers of the psyche. Somewhere hidden in early development a decision was made that this internal experience is unbearable or unacceptable, and must be discarded. To reclaim it, it is thought, would be dangerous. Yet to keep it hidden requires defenses that may be creating problems.

THE NEED FOR A THEORY OF AFFECT, EMOTION, AND FEELING

To study defenses it is necessary to understand the various experiences that are being defended against. Unfortunately, psychological theory as yet lacks a fully developed systematic theory of affect, emotion, and feeling, and these terms continue to be used almost interchangeably (Basch, 1983; Green, 1977; Rapaport, 1967). While there has been extensive work on the development of cognition and language, until recently a theoretical study of the affect-emotion-feeling triad has been relatively neglected. Since these elements are basic to all behavior, the absence of an integrated theory hampers our understanding of human behavior and motivation.

Attempts to develop a theory of affect have led to various formulations. Freud described a division of the mind in terms of "process." The critical dualism was *not* between affects and thought, but between two types of thinking, including primary and secondary process (Freud, 1911). Affectivity as the first element of the triad precedes the development of thinking processes. Affect is the earliest psychological experience in response to the child's interaction with the world (Basch, 1983), and provides another mode of interpersonal communication. Jones (1984) posits that affects are a language, a nonreflective coding process for receiving and processing information. Kerr and Bowen (1988) distinguish between human beings who are capable of expressing feelings and species of animals that experience emotions such as rage, fear, and disgust, but do not possess thinking, language or feelings. "The feeling and intellectual systems are fairly recent acquisitions in the evolutionary line of animals that led to *homo sapiens*. When these systems were added and developed during the gradual course of human evolution, they did not replace, except perhaps partially, the functions of the emotional system" (Kerr and Bowen, p. 31).

ELEMENTS OF THE TRIAD AND THE USE OF DEFENSES

Figure 5.1 gives examples of a few of the building blocks of internal experiences that color an individual's personal view of the world. These include feelings, emotions and, at the most archaic level, affects. Varying mixtures of internal reactions, lack of control, confusion and anxiety result in a series of defenses to protect the vulnerable self. These defenses correspond to the ability to contain the arousal of the elements of the triad without the need to immediately ward it off. In more pathological states, feelings and emotions are characteristically passed over and the defenses operate at more regressed affective level.

Every developmental phase incorporates the previous ones with responses to new experiences integrating some aspect of the old interactive dynamics. "Each adds a new dimension to the comprehension of affective communication, encompassing and integrating what has gone before, without, however, eliminating the possibility of a response at earlier levels" (Basch, 1983, p. 117).

The infant comes into the world prepared to relate to others and is sensitive to affective communications of others from the beginning of life (Burlingham, 1967; Stern, 1985). As the child moves through a series of developmental steps to adulthood, internal experiences may include

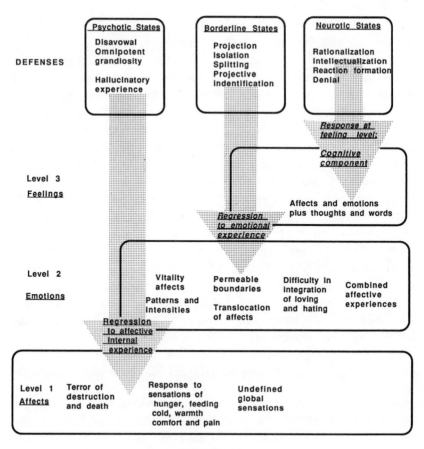

FIGURE 5.1
The Emotional System Basis of Defenses

affective states, emotional reactions, and combinations of complex feelings. What is needed is a clear and precise understanding of the difference between the internal experiences of affectivity, emotionality, and feeling, how each develops in terms of early life history and how they combine with cognition. I begin with some definitions that clarify my views of the affectual-emotional-feeling system and related defensive reactions.

Affects are basic to the organization of experience and to the development of a "core self" (Stern, 1985) during the early months of life. A limited repertoire of affects is present from birth, or even before. These are undefined global sensations related to experiences with bodily functions, physical comfort or pain in nurturing, and/or deprivation experiences between infant and caretaker. They are based on the purely affective reactions of the infant to hunger, cold, pain, and a host of not yet defined sensations experienced by the infant. Initially these affective responses are automatic reactions to the frequency, intensity, and rate of increase or decrease of stimulation. At first they are not psychological events but purely biological responses. However, they quickly become linked to encoded memory traces and become the building blocks of emotions and feelings.

In adults "affective sensation is processed so rapidly that consciousness of what has taken place comes after the fact" (Basch, 1983, p. 115). As a result of this rapidity, adults experiencing an affective response often do not know how to recognize its emergence or specify the reason for its occurrence. Without awareness of its presence, affectivity penetrates life events.

Tomkins (1980) notes that affects are contagious and tend to influence those who are in near proximity. Sadness or anxiety felt by a mother results in very similar affective reactions in a child. Also, specific states, such as rage, tend to generalize to "any person coming within our orbit, . . . to satisfy the need to express" (Clynes, 1980, p. 297). More often those who are in our orbit are family members. The most vulnerable members become the receivers of undigested, "spit out" affects.

Emotions are responses that incorporate patterns of seeing, hearing, smelling and touching, with varying intensity and vitality of experience. Emotional responses are formed during interactional experiences that include some awareness of self and other. Before the infant has developed the ability to symbolize or organize thoughts into words, powerful sensations and affects combined with awareness of reactions from others are being processed and responded to emotionally.

Affects and emotions each vary in depth and intensity. The infant may be happy or sad, very happy, or deeply sad. Emotions are generalized and act as a focus or template when new experiences draw into awareness earlier experiences that are in memory (Clynes, 1980). It is in these more complex emotional patterns that we may experience ourselves as related, unrelated, or negatively related to others in our environment. Generalized emotion, then, is basic to development of an internalized representation of the world of self and others.

Feelings combine emotions and affects with cognitive processes. When a degree of conscious thought is added to affect, emotion and feelings are available to awareness. When the infant becomes capable of symbolic ability, "the conscious awareness of an affective event as a subjective experience that we call a 'feeling' becomes a possibility" (Basch, 1983, p. 117). This generally occurs by the age of 18 to 24 months when language develops and feelings can be expressed in words. An emerging vocabulary gives the developing child opportunities to choose whether or not to share inner experience.

Feelings involve intellectual awareness of the outermost layer of the emotional system. Employing cognitive capacity and language, feelings are of a higher order than raw affect or emotion. While the developmental step of using feelings to identify and name affect is possible as the infant reaches certain capacities, it is not inevitable. Defenses may interfere by suppressing or ejecting them from conscious awareness.

Although awareness of affects, emotions, and feelings may be cut off, nothing is lost. Thus, regressions to affective or emotional states are likely to occur in interactions at various times in life. Since rationality is highly valued in human beings, there is a tendency to utilize language to explain whatever is experienced internally in as logical a sequence as possible. To most people, what is irrational is considered crazy. To "lose your mind" is equated with being out of control, to be mad, or go insane. The reemergence of primitive affect and precognitive emotionality is, therefore, generally guarded against.

EXPERIENCES THAT MUST BE DEFENDED AGAINST

In Figure 5.2 we see that from a level 1 affective perspective defenses guard against a core fear of annihilation anxiety and the experience of self-fragmentation. These fears, related to damage to the sense of self, are the most archaic. Oedipal fears that develop by the third year of life are "secondary to the indescribable core annihilation fear" (Cooper, 1986, p. 116). When the need to maintain a cohesive and developing self is thwarted, a variety of anxieties and protective measures is set in motion.

Between level 1 and level 2 there is an intermediary developmental experience. Transitional objects (Winnicott, 1965) such as a security blanket are utilized to navigate between the internal world of fantasy, need fulfillment, and affectivity, on the one hand, and the interpersonal world of self and others, on the other.

As the infant becomes more cognizant of and reactive to the environment, new awareness can evoke major narcissistic wounds, causing intense anxiety early in life. Among these are the discovery of otherness, the discovery of sexual differences, and the discovery of mortality (McDougall, 1986). Each of these is an occasion for trauma. A fourth terrifying discovery is suggested by Chasseguet-Smirgel (1984) – the awareness of the difference in power and size between the young child and those older and larger than himself.

As the developing child becomes increasingly facile in the use of language and modes of interactive communications, primary affective responses become symbolized, identified in words, and sometimes experi-

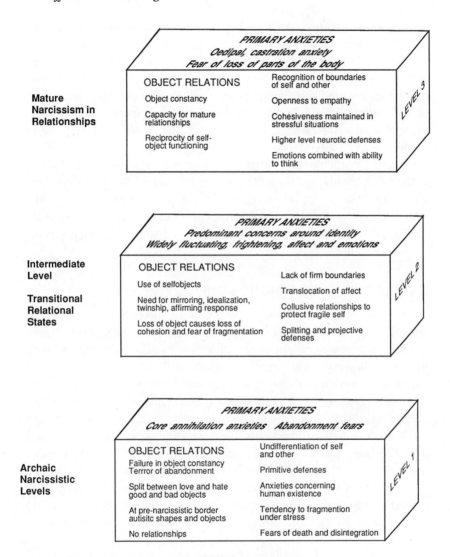

FIGURE 5.2

Narcissistic Structures in Relationships

enced in opposition to each other. At this time one feeling state may be mobilized to defend against another. The child wishing to please the mother and attain her love and devotion may simultaneously wish to assert an independent action and fear the power of the mother's disapproval. The feared reaction may be so anxiety-provoking that cognitive processes fail to function. Only the earlier dread of destruction is experienced at that moment.

As another example, the child who observes an alcoholic father beat a crying, cringing mother may assume culpability for the discord and make a decision to always be "good." A lifetime of goodness hides awareness of the frightening internal experience whenever problems arise. The emotions may be experienced as so dangerous that an unconscious decision is made to feel nothing. Alternatively, the child may view mother as weak and vulnerable and father's aggressiveness as strength, and determine never to become weak or defenseless.

At level 3 of the developmental process there is a recognition of others as separate, an awareness of boundaries of self, and an ability to combine affectivity with cognitive awareness. Intersubjective relatedness includes affect attunement and the mutual sharing of affective states (Stolorow et al., 1987). Without such relational attunement, activities are solitary, private, and idiosyncratic (Basch, 1985).

DEVELOPMENT OF BORDERLINE DEFENSES

Borderline defenses have their precursors in the somewhat more advanced but still very archaic stage of the infant's development during the first year of life. They have to do not only with emerging affectivity, but also with patterns of interactions and reactions related to fluctuations in a caretaker's response and with uncertainty about expected reactions that become generalized and experienced as dangerous or affectually overwhelming to the developing self of the child. Confusing responses and dual affectual experiences result in a precarious convergence of self and environment. Affects may combine, conflict, or augment each other in the development of emotions. This occurs at a point even before full awareness of self and other. Pleasurable and unpleasurable emotions may become dichotomized and confused as the infant reacts to a mother's presence after an overlong delay in responding. The splitting of frightening emotions characterizes many borderline defenses.

After there is a recognition of separateness of self and other, and a beginning ability to recognize that there are important needs met by caretaking figures, the emotions evoked by perceived failures in parental responsiveness give rise to a different kind of defensive pattern. The infant develops awareness that an emotional display influences parents' reactions. Cognition and affectivity sometimes combine, with the intent of obtaining desired outcomes. Sometimes the developing child learns that the inner self must be distorted in order to obtain needed emotional and physical provisions. The decision to distort produces a series of neurotic-narcissistic defenses.

PATTERNS OF DEFENSIVE RESPONSE

In the imagined interactions of Martha and Harry described in Chapter 3, the alternative possibilities demonstrate the differences in the ways that various levels of defense may be acted out in a relationship. Reactions may be a regression to unthinking, screaming infancy. Alternatively, there may be an upsetting experience that is combined with a cognitive awareness of the other person's needs and feelings.

In any individual there are defensive fluctuations according to the current environmental situation. Nevertheless, there is a tendency to regress to predetermined patterns of defensive response in times of high anxiety or stress. We will look at some of these patterns in detail.

Splitting Love and Hate

Splitting occurs as the child comes to believe there are "bad" things inside that must be gotten rid of. These are split off from awareness. They may be consciously forgotten and not allowed to grow or develop. They survive but are denied and hidden away in the unconscious. Such feelings may include envy, hatred, fear of dependency, loss of identity, etc. Love and rage, good and bad, may become polarized, with only one or the other allowed into consciousness. Much energy must be directed toward keeping these feelings from coming into conscious awareness and finding places to lodge them safely.

Where splitting is a prominent defense, idealized love may suddenly turn to hate. Ordinarily, hate-filled images are kept out of consciousness, with the intent of preserving the good and loving. However, when there is massive disappointment in another, an opportunity to "dump" the negative feelings emerges. In the process of splitting, even where there is no evidence of severe pathology, some dangers may arise. The inner self is split off from awareness, with a tremendous investment in the "false self," a facade of functionality presented as a bulwark of self-worth and isolated from any threatening emotions.

Projective Identification

Related to splitting, projective identification (Klein, 1946; Kernberg, 1975; Grotstein, 1981; Ogden, 1982) may cause feelings to be psychologically relocated into others in near proximity. The process of splitting and concurrent projective identification is one of the earliest of the defenses and is designed to protect against overwhelming affect as the emergent self develops. When this defense pattern is utilized, there is a need to exert active control over the other in order to evade feelings of danger or of hopelessness (Grotstein, 1981).

Projective identification is a script that is played by two. The process involves psychologically transferring a piece of oneself into another and then inducing the other to behave in accordance with the projection. In severe pathological conditions there is the fantasy of putting into another unacceptable negative affects and emotions; then, the dangerous other must be defended against. It is upsetting and frightening to see one's inner emotions and hateful images—too awful to acknowledge in oneself—now residing in another. At the same time, the recipient of these negative affects is a person who is very close. The holder of these dangerous and destructive feelings is perceived to be in a position to throw them back in a hostile attack. It is in such a situation that we sometimes see couples who cannot tolerate each other because they carry each other's most unacceptable and intolerable qualities. At the same time, they cannot part because they serve the function of carrying these unacceptable qualities for each other. There is a need to keep the other close and to maintain control at all times.

The following scenario exemplifies the projection and transfer of emotional upset from one spouse to another. Gus has learned that he was passed over for a promotion. He does not wish to tell his wife, Helga, because she is always comparing him unfavorably to the husbands of her sisters. He feels pangs of failure, and experiences stress and anxiety. At that moment Helga walks into the room. Gus greets her by asking where she put the nails that he needs to repair the stairs. Helga says she does not know where the nails are. "Why can't I ever find anything in this house? Why do you put things where they cannot be found?" he demands of her. "I must fix those stairs now, before someone falls and breaks a leg. I need you to go out and buy the nails while I start working on the stairs right now." To this Helga replies, "But it's almost 6 p.m. The stores will be closed. Besides, I've got to make dinner." "I said that I need it now. If you hurry you can get there before the store closes," he says. Helga does not wish to do what her husband wants and says angrily, "I'm tired, and you were using the nails last weekend. You must have put them somewhere. If you can't find them you go out to get some more," she tells him. He shouts at her, "You never do anything to help me, you bitch." "Goddamn you," she screams. "I wish I had never married you." "Feel free to leave if you wish. Who needs you anyway? You never do anything around here. Why don't you get out?" he fires at her in rapid succession. "You can cook your own dinner," she says tearfully as she runs into the bedroom and slams the door. "There she goes, always crying. All I was trying to do is fix the house for her and she starts a fight over nothing."

Helga finds herself in their recurrent marital dilemma—either do exactly as her husband demands or fight with him. Tired and upset, she withdraws from the predicament in frustrated rage. The tension that Gus felt earlier dissipates as Helga is entrapped in this collusive interchange. It is she, rather than he, who now experiences the turmoil. "It's hard to live with such a crazy lady," he says to himself, calmly turning on the television. "I wonder why I put up with her." This couple's mode of living together has a component of pathological projective identification and a reciprocal taking in of renounced affectivity.

Translocation of Shared Affectivity

In projective identification there is an unconscious fantasy of translocating aspects of the self into the internal mental image of another. The self tries to rid itself of its unwanted, split-off parts or to share emotions for which words are unavailable. Although generally considered pathological processes, the internal experiences of splitting and projective identification are fairly universal, occurring not only in pathological form, but also "in all of us in less intense form" (Grotstein, 1981, p. 252). Differentiation of self and other is required for projection to be actively employed (Stolorow and Lachmann, 1980).

The process originates as an attempt to share archaic affects that took form before there were words, and continues in hidden form until something in adult life triggers the experience anew. Another person is enlisted to accept, understand, and contain the primitive emotional reactions. Indeed, when the individual believes that he or she has found such a person, it is natural to "communicate" with that person through a process of translocation of affectivity.

If the infant-maternal bond was such that messages of affectivity, even very frightening or painful ones, were understood and benignly responded to, then there is a generalized legacy of emotional attunement. This responsiveness will be carried into adult relationships. When one partner in a relationship lives through another or idealizes the other and takes great pleasure in shining in the other's reflected glory, boundaries are temporarily removed. The mate, in complementary fashion, accepts what is translocated and responds in a way that enhances the self-esteem or emotional security of both partners. This is a defensive pattern that can provide the key to a mutually adaptive relationship.

Dual Track Thinking

Most individuals in conflict or under stress maintain a rational part of themselves that keeps them from losing control of their actions, even when overwhelming emotions affect them. The ability to stand back and monitor one's own participation allows for the emergence of an "observing ego." At the same time, it is not unusual for relatively undisturbed individuals, "normal neurotics" (that is, most of us), to carry within them certain pockets of pathology (Klein, 1981) and to occasionally experience episodes during which the observing ego is lost.

The human mind functions on several tracks at the same time (Grotstein, 1981). It is possible to be murderously enraged without murdering another. It is possible to be erotically aroused toward another without acting sexually. It is possible to participate emotionally in an experience with others, while at the same time standing back and observing the experience. It is possible to think and feel at the same time if one is not frightened that immersion in the emotional experience will be overwhelming. It is possible to accuse another of being the cause of one's distress even while recognizing that the target of reproach actually was not to blame. Only when the mind totally distorts the events in the interaction does the projected attack completely deny the reality of the other.

Lansky (1985) speculates that when partners are totally lost in blaming or attacking transactions, they are in a special ego state, different from their usual state of mind. In this state, the "observing ego" is unavailable for conscious reflection on the process while it is happening. The ego state that attacks or provokes attack is unavailable to reasoning or to other states of consciousness. Thus, attacking prevents not only resolution of the immediate issues but also the emergence of other material. In a more rational state of conscious awareness, one or both battling partners may be ashamed of or bewildered by their attacking behavior.

Darin's case exemplifies such "dual track thinking." In the day-to-day life of his marriage, he seems quite capable of interacting rationally, discussing differences, hearing what his wife Jennifer says. Darin is quite adequate in reasonable problem-solving. However, in stressful situations, when the dual track states of consciousness emerge, he is not only unable to communicate rationally, but also hardly aware of Jennifer's existence. When the outburst of anger is over, he reverts to the status quo. Furthermore, he refuses to discuss with Jennifer what happened. Each time one of Darin's outbursts occurs, Jennifer pulls away a little emotionally. At the same time, Darin seems so calm, so normal and reasonable, that she is left with the thought that it was simply an aberration that will never occur again. It is beyond her understanding, but she has said in therapy that one day she will snap and just turn him off. If that happens, she says, she will leave him. If she does, Darin will not understand why. His mechanisms of splitting off the rage and suppressing the memory protect him from knowing how it feels to live with the anger that boils up inside.

Indeed, while spouses may function at a fairly mature level outside the relationship, they still may encourage attacking interactions within the marriage in order to get rid of traits they would like to disown. Attacking interactions go beyond locating culpability in the partner instead of oneself. In part, they constitute an attack on activities that threaten the couple's bond. Attacking interactions are used to cover neediness, extreme dependency, and low self-esteem.

NARROW EMOTIONAL RANGE IN NARCISSISTIC VULNERABILITY

There are adults whose emotional range runs the gamut from A to A. They feel nothing, show little emotional reaction but at times explode in anger. Afterward they have difficulty understanding what provoked such an intense reaction. Defenses against chronic emptiness may include an attempt to escape through frantic involvement in professional or social activities or by inappropriate utilization of sex, food, alcohol, or drugs.

Sometimes thwarted emotionality leads to various internal and interactional compensations and psychosomatic process. What the mind cannot allow into consciousness is experienced somatically (McDougall, 1985). When defenses become impaired or do not regulate well, physical symptoms can develop (Brenner, 1974, 1975). Emotions may thus be internalized and somaticized, or externalized in disguised fashion (McDougall, 1986, p. 153). Suppressed affect may be converted into hysterical symptoms, displaced onto a new representation, or turned into obsessions, overwhelming anxiety reactions, or physical problems.

MUTUALLY SUPPORTIVE COLLUSIONS

In psychotherapy there is an attempt to permit a person to re-admit elements of the self that have been split off, so that he or she can reinstate and consciously experience a feeling of wholeness. The therapist accepts the "bad," split-off part of the self that is experienced as so toxic by the patient and, in the process of understanding, accepting and not finding it intolerable, is able to detoxify the "badness" before giving it back in the form of conscious awareness.

Often, what patients do with therapists, partners do with each other. They use projective defenses in an attempt to get the partner to accept feelings that cannot be described or tolerated. The unconscious wish of each partner in an intimate relationship is that the other will provide an arena of safety, a healing function. One of the greatest joys of lovers is their intense sharing of their inner selves. Often new love is a process of testing the extent to which the intimate other can understand and accept aspects that are barely known to the self. In the closeness of a marriage or an intimate relationship, difficulties arise, over the long run, when partners fail to accept important aspects of each other.

Marital collusions are an attempt between mates to recreate the interactions of an earlier relationship. Such collusions occur in the hope that this time the needs will be responded to and the self will be affirmed, thus newly activating arrested growth. Sometimes this works. Sometimes it results in endless battles.

Each participant in the unconscious collusion (Willi, 1982) has an investment in maintaining it. Each spouse accepts the projection of the other's unwanted aspects and comes to act in ways that confirm the partner's expectations. The spouses' defensive structures mesh and stabilize. Narcissistic collusions built on mutual defenses are aimed at protecting the individual, the partnership, and the family from those remnants of early experience perceived as so potentially destructive that they must be disguised, denied, and put out of awareness. How that can work to the mutual benefit of each partner can be seen in the case of Sally and Reggie, whose relationship was described in Chapter 3.

DEFENSIVE COLLUSIONS

There are marriages that are organized around containment and the collusive exchange of projective defenses to avoid some nameless dread, such as the terror of abandonment or destructive fantasies. A pattern of interactional events that causes reemergence of early fears of being left helpless and unable to provide for urgent needs can result in debilitating anxiety and the possibility of fragmentation. In such situations there is often an entitled, demanding rageful insistence on justice that goes beyond specific issues. Each spouse, of course, sees the difficulties as emanating from the other. To the partners, real communication is a danger, not an opportunity to improve the situation, because of their fear of exposure and humiliation (Lansky, 1981, 1985).

These couples may regard their marriage as a disaster, often to such an extent that they are unable to explain even to themselves why they remain attached to a partner who is apparently so despicable. They cannot understand why their attacking marriages have endured despite decades of unremitting misery.

Don and Donna

This pattern is evident in the marriage of Don and Donna, who have complaints going back to the beginning of their marriage. Donna says that her husband is rigid, controlling, and emotionally unavailable. Don complains that this wife would rather do anything—be at work, talk on the telephone with her friends, take a class, or play with their son—rather than spend any time with him. He tries not to get angry at her lack of attention, but it enrages him that she has so much to give to everyone else and so little for him. Once in a while he tells her that he is upset; she then reacts as though he has physically attacked her. She becomes so tearful and upset that he simply gives up and withdraws.

Don's reactions are understandable in the context of his early relationships. Don had a depressed mother who eventually died of an overdose of pills. Although the doctors said the death was accidental, he believes that his mother became so distressed with their marginal life and financial situation that she killed herself. As an adult, Don put his entire emotional energy into achieving the financial success that makes a luxurious lifestyle possible for him and his family. He is not satisfied that he has done enough and secretly believes that that is why his wife is seldom there for him emotionally or sexually.

Donna, meanwhile, has no idea why Don avoided her when she was going through periods of great emotional turmoil, including the death of her mother and her own life-threatening illness. In relationships with female friends she gives herself freely. She wants and gets a similar emotional response from her friends. She is angry and frustrated that her husband does not seem to have the capacity to let down his defenses enough to "play with me" and "be with me." She also reports being frightened of him when he seems angry but denies what she sees.

Examination of Donna's family history reveals a father who abused her physically and emotionally, and who was abused himself as an orphaned immigrant child. When he became enraged, Donna fled in fear of his beatings, often locking herself in the bathroom, where she trembled with fear. Any sign of anger, therefore, causes her to withdraw. Both husband and wife desperately seek contact. Each blames the other for its absence.

Don and Donna need to move from a destructive collusion to an adaptive one. What they need is a path through which each may come to empathically understand the needs, fears and defensive patterns of the other. As each recognizes that the long-held patterns of their relationship are designed to protect their damaged selves from further injury, they may slowly begin to let down their barriers against each other. In the process both must increase their tolerance for anxiety when events cause the emergence of previously frightening or dangerous affects.

Ann and Jim

Ann and Jim are both successful in their careers, working 12 to 14 hours a day. Jim is also trying to write a novel. They seem the perfect pair, and their friends and acquaintances envy them and their lifestyle. Ann makes friends easily, and Jim entertains them well and keeps them interested once Ann has made contact. Nevertheless, their life and work schedules keep them from having very much intimate emotional or sexual contact with each other.

On those rare occasions when they do manage to connect, Ann fills the air with her definite ideas about how Jim should dress and how the house should be run and how their lovemaking should go. She sees herself as giving simple suggestions that would make their life together more comfortable. If he loved her, she explains, he would want to do these things for her. Ann needs a great deal of reassurance that Jim loves her. The result is that the only acceptable way for Jim to prove his love is to do things exactly her way.

Jim thinks that Ann is trying to control him. Not only that, but whatever he does, it is not enough to satisfy Ann. As soon as Jim experiences Ann as demanding, he feels anger well up, just as in childhood the anger began to well up in response to his father's demandingness. He feels the anger arising when Ann tries to initiate lovemaking. He withholds, avoids, withdraws, becomes impotent and very upset, and goes from being extremely rational to experiencing himself as a deflated, empty and enraged child. Jim is torn between guilt and anger. The two of them handle their feelings now by not seeing very much of each other.

Ann's view of the world is one that portrays her constantly as a victim, which makes it difficult for her to discriminate her own thoughts, wishes, and intentions from those of her husband. Her demands convey an underlying desire to replicate a fantasy of "perfect" symbiotic fusion. In this relationship, Jim is supposed to perform exactly as she would. When he "fails" her, she comes face to face with her own chaotic internal self or becomes depressed and fragmented. Thus, he must be available when she needs him, to soothe her and confirm that she is indeed a whole and loveable human being.

At the same time, Jim is not simply a victim of Ann's unreasonable needs. He has his own reasons for maintaining this relationship. He is part of a mutual pattern of identifications, internalizations and defensive collusions. To Jim, Ann is a recreation of the father who would walk in on his peaceful reading and attack him for not taking the garbage out or not raking the lawn. He carries a feeling of both rage and guilt — rage because he never knew when or why he would be hurt by his father's outbursts and guilt because he secretly believed that he had done something to cause his father to be so upset with him. In treatment he came to recognize that he still believed that he was causing Ann's anger. He also felt that somehow he had a chance to change the pattern. He was trying to heal old wounds by curing Ann of her tendency to blow up at him.

EFFECT ON RELATIONSHIPS

When there is a history of narcissistic vulnerability, partners join together to protect themselves and each other from conflict. A collusive contract maintains the consistency of each partner's perceptions. In that way, neither is forced to deal with overwhelming negative feelings about oneself. By masking pathology and blending it with the present intimate other, narcissistic collusion often creates merely a joyless semblance of safety and security, not a haven of comfort and love.

Attempts at collusion tend to develop into pathological symptoms. Ongoing interactions reinforce the collusion by allowing each of the mates to maintain an archaic inner world that the other projectively supports. The behavior of each spouse is needed to confirm the other's distorted view of reality, while the collusion is necessary to keep destructive inner forces at bay within each of the partners. Any change in the system reactivates defensive rather than adaptive mechanisms (Nadelson and Paolino, 1978).

Depending upon what dangerous or painful feelings are locked away, the defenses that are meant to protect the vulnerable self from being overwhelmed by the triad of affect or emotion or feeling may be acted out or turned inward, causing damage to the body, to the psyche, and to close relationships. When archaic affectivity reemerges, boundaries between self and other are in danger of being transgressed through archaic defenses such as splitting and projective identification. Boundaries may then be put up as a barrier to avoid being overwhelmed from without and to protect from dangers of uncontrolled states within. Choices are made throughout life either to defend against unacceptable or intolerable affects and emotions or to attempt to repair the early damage and reintegrate the feelings. The degree to which affects, emotions, and feelings can be held and contained without use of defenses is an important part of emotional well-being. The ability of mates to function as containers to hold the vulnerable self of the other in times of need, stress, or frustration has important implications for the well-being of the relationship.

Part Two of this book examines these issues further and presents a model for understanding and changing troubled relationships.

PART TWO

CHAPTER 6

Presenting Problems and Underlying Problems

Issues of the therapeutic dyad, including transference, resistance, defense mechanisms and empathy, have received much scrutiny in the psychodynamic literature. But dyadic relationships are not limited to interactions between patient and therapist; the very same forces operate in any intimate relationship. Just as thoughts, feelings and actions that occur in an analytic session are often derivatives of underlying psychological issues, marital complaints reflect core individual themes. When a marital problem is identified, the therapeutic tasks are to discover the inner meaning and motivating behavior underlying the presenting issues and to clarify relationship dynamics that affect the psychological functioning of the individuals involved.

There is a wide variety of presenting problems. Among the many issues people are known to fight about, Blumstein and Schwartz (1983) investigated money, work and sex, which are assumed to be the basis of most marital difficulties. After many years of treating couples I am convinced that the issues that most couples believe cause their unhappiness are only the outer casing, a kernel of truth that provides a rationale for discontent in the relationship. Underlying these identified problems are individual issues of narcissistic vulnerability and mutually activated collusions that protect each person from the emergence of overwhelming affectivity.

In this chapter, I will illustrate with case histories my contention that a host of presenting problems have a narrow base of underlying causes—narcissistic vulnerability and injuries to self-image. Fundamental to many identified relationship problems are issues of power and control, independence and dependence, closeness and distance. More often than not, couples at first do not even recognize that there are issues other than the crisis that has brought them to treatment. Deeply hidden wounds to self-esteem may make it impossible for the partners to reach agreement about anything.

To make changes in the functional relationship between the spouses, overt and covert behavior patterns must be modified. This may be done by developing new habits of interaction, by helping them gain new insight, or through particular paradoxical interventions that provoke change. Generally, a question about what needs problem behaviors serve will elicit responses about clearly understood issues of money, work, and sex or about the expectations each has of the other and of the relationship.

An important part of the early assessment process is understanding the way each partner has learned to be in the world, including the recreation of early developmental experiences, and how their hopes and expectations of relationships cause a joint interactional process that results in their particular relationship. A partner's view may be presented as, "He is driving me to drink," or "She pushed me, so I pushed her back. I didn't mean to hurt her." An examination of the implied provocations may elicit information on the mutually collusive aspects of the partnership and news about the deeper underlying individual fantasies and fears that each carries into any intimate relationship. Here we come to understand the kinds of reactions that are specific to their interactions and those behaviors that might emerge no matter to whom the partners were married.

For some people, a hug not given, a phone call not returned, a birthday or anniversary forgotten is experienced as a major rejection. They either become angry or withdraw, a fight-flight reaction (Bion, 1961). If the partner is similarly vulnerable, the relationship will break down or will be experienced as walking on eggs and occasionally stepping on a grenade.

The understanding of what is occurring in a relationship is somewhat like an archeological excavation in which we begin with the surface features and soon uncover various layers of mutual problems and resources. Figure 6.1 gives a visual representation of the kinds of simultaneous problems that are occurring at the point where people come into therapy.

We have come to recognize that symptoms that were formed early in the lives of either or both spouses can appear later in life in a renewed attempt to resolve old issues. Couples may join together to protect themselves and each other from inner conflict. A collusive contract maintains the consistency of each partner's perceptions. In this way, neither must deal with overwhelming negative or dangerous emotions. Unfortunately, reciprocity of

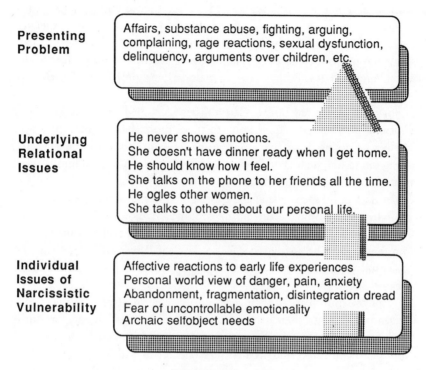

Presenting Problem

Affairs, substance abuse, fighting, arguing, complaining, rage reactions, sexual dysfunction, delinquency, arguments over children, etc.

Underlying Relational Issues

He never shows emotions.
She doesn't have dinner ready when I get home.
He should know how I feel.
She talks on the phone to her friends all the time.
He ogles other women.
She talks to others about our personal life.

Individual Issues of Narcissistic Vulnerability

Affective reactions to early life experiences
Personal world view of danger, pain, anxiety
Abandonment, fragmentation, disintegration dread
Fear of uncontrollable emotionality
Archaic selfobject needs

FIGURE 6.1
Presenting Problems and Underlying Issues

this type can do little more than provide a temporary illusion of comfort. More often, what is created are new symptoms: the mental or physical dysfunction of one or both mates, a sexual or emotional relationship with an outside person, or a child's acting-out. By masking pathology and blending it with whatever mature love is present, narcissistic collusion is often merely a joyless semblance of safety and security, not a haven of comfort and love.

Joan and Peter

Recently I was called for a consultation by a woman who had an urgent dilemma. She was three months into a pregnancy and could not decide whether to have the baby or get an abortion. Her lover, the father of the baby, suggested that he could come in with her, as the decision was important to him also. As the sessions unfolded, it became clear that at issue were not only questions about the pregnancy and their relationship, but also many areas of vulnerability in each of them. Peter vacillated between two women as a way of gratifying a need for acceptance and affirmation that seemed greater than either his wife or girlfriend could fill. Joan, desperately seeking love, consistently formed alliances with men like her father— unable to commit to anyone. The following description of my first session with Peter and Joan shows how the underlying problems of each mate emerge in the therapeutic session with a couple.

Joan and Peter are in their late thirties. Although Peter has a wife in Chicago, his business requires him to travel more than six months a year. He began dating Joan over four years ago and, although he felt great attraction to her, he had no intention of becoming seriously committed to a relationship. But he found himself increasingly involved, and once they began dating, he spent less and less time in Chicago. Joan was nearing the age when she would be unable to conceive. Although she was a senior executive in a cosmetics firm, the urge to have a baby had become stronger in recent years. She attributed it to her love for Peter and her wish to have his child. After they talked about getting married for some time, she became pregnant.

Over the four years of their relationship many problems had developed that interfered with their plans to marry. Peter lost his job and was out of work for six months. He became restless and easily angered. He took calls from Cathy, his wife, and seemed very concerned with Cathy's health and state of mind. Joan became increasingly frustrated and wondered if he would ever marry her. Now she had told Peter that if they were not getting married quickly she would have an abortion. Peter indicated that he very much wanted her to have his baby and did intend to marry her, but something always seemed to get in the way of their plans to have a wedding.

When Joan called for an appointment she requested help in clarifying the situation and in making decisions about the relationship and about having the baby. What emerged in the session was much more complicated than the question of marriage.

> THERAPIST Can you tell me why you are here?
>
> JOAN I came here to see you because I am wondering what to do about this relationship that I have with Peter. I don't know what to do about getting married, or what to do about my pregnancy.
>
> THERAPIST You say you came in, Joan. Peter is here also, although you were the one who made the appointment.
>
> JOAN Last night, when we were real affectionate, I told Peter that I was coming here. He thought it might be a good idea if we came to- gether. But this morning, he looked as though he was being forced.

THERAPIST   How do you feel about being here, Peter?

PETER   It's fine with me, although I don't know why we can't just talk to each other. I believe in laying our cards out on the table and solving our problems. It's not a Chinese puzzle where we need translators. I don't know why Joan thought we needed someone outside to tell us what to do. If she does, that may be another problem that will concern me.

THERAPIST   You believe that you should be strong enough to figure out what is wrong and resolve it without someone outside telling you the answers.

JOAN   We tried that and it didn't work. We've still got problems. We have to resolve them, especially now that I have to decide what to do about the baby.

THERAPIST   Are you concerned about whether or not to marry or is the question related to the pregnancy?

JOAN   It has to do with our whole relationship, not the pregnancy but the whole relationship needs work.

PETER   I don't like your blaming me for getting pregnant. It's not like a shotgun wedding. You knew what you were doing.

THERAPIST   Tell me what the situation is with the relationship and how being pregnant fits in.

JOAN   Peter is married. His wife will never let him go. My family is not happy because of our religious differences and the fact that he was getting a divorce. Now, he has gone ahead and filed for divorce and we're talking about marriage.

PETER   It used to be real good together. Now I think we have to resolve our problems before we go ahead and marry or bring a child into the world.

THERAPIST   You seem to be talking about different issues. Maybe we'd better look more closely at what has gone wrong—how you each see it. Can you start by telling me how it was when this relationship began?

JOAN   Four years ago, we were both working for [a large multinational corporation] requiring a lot of travel by employees. Peter was traveling in England, France, and throughout the United States. We only saw each other on business occasions. Then we began going out together after work. By the third time we met, Peter said he was madly in love with me. From then on, when he was in town, we were constantly together. We had a wonderful relationship. I never pushed for it, but Peter very quickly said he wanted to marry me. But he was still married to Cathy. They had been married for 13 years. He told me that he would divorce her and we could get married. But his wife put every obstacle in the way. She has a heart condition, and she uses his guilt to hold onto him. She clung to him. She kept calling him. He started the divorce proceedings but never finished them. Then he lost his job. He was out of work for six months. I kept thinking that was what was making him so depressed and upset. He always seemed to be upset with me. But we were determined to be together. Meanwhile, Cathy continued to make problems for us. The day we moved in together, Cathy sent a dozen roses with a message to me as though it was a lover of mine, trying to make me look cheap. She keeps calling Peter, begging him to come back.

Peter sat and watched Joan talk about him but said nothing and hardly moved a muscle. I was aware that I was hardly moving a muscle myself and felt a great deal of tension at that moment in the session. I recognized that I had to separate my own values and thoughts about what they were saying to me from what might be going on between the two of them.

THERAPIST How did you react to this?

JOAN I thought she would stop but she never did. I felt sorry for Peter. He was too guilty about leaving a sick wife to tell her to stop. Sometimes he would call her back or go to see her. He always came back to me. Then, in September, he said we should get married. He wanted us to have a baby and he cut up my diaphragm. A friend of mine even offered to let us use her house for the wedding. It was a perfect setting. When I told Peter about it, I saw he was not as excited as I was. He said we were having too many arguments and it was not like it used to be. We didn't get married, but we still were not using contraceptives. I told Peter to be careful during my monthly cycle when I could get pregnant. One night, when we were away on vacation, I warned him to pull out but he didn't. That's why I blame him.

THERAPIST It makes you very upset that first Peter wanted you to get pregnant and now that you are pregnant he seems to be hesitating about marrying you. So you need to decide what to do—whether you and Peter will get married, and if not, whether or not to have the baby.

Peter, do you have any thoughts on this or any reaction to what Joan said?

PETER Well, she got it right with some modifications. Our relationship used to be wonderful. I don't know what went wrong. Joan always seems so upset. I feel pulled by Cathy. I'm not sure about marriage now and I don't know what to think about Joan's having an abortion, I guess she should if we aren't getting married.

JOAN   I don't want to raise our baby alone. I used to think your short temper was because you were out of work for such a long time. Now, you're back at work and you still get upset. You still take Cathy's phone calls. You even go out to call and talk to her.

(Turning to the therapist) When he goes out somewhere, I just know he's going to call her. If I ask, he tells me the truth.

THERAPIST   (Turning back to their immediate problem) Joan, you called for a consultation to help you decide whether or not to continue with the pregnancy, but as you and Peter talk it is obvious that there is much more going on that you have to decide. First, you both seem to agree that you don't want to bring a child into the world unless you work out your relationship together. You have some serious concerns about the nature of your relationship. Joan, from the form you filled out I see that you are close to 40. You may be worried about your biological clock, and wondering if this is your last chance to have a baby. Also, your relationship seems to be at some kind of an impasse. Peter, you seem to want Joan to be the way she was when you first met—alive, totally involved with you—and you are disappointed when she is not there for you emotionally. Joan, it is hard to be there in a positive emotional way when you are angry that Peter isn't keeping his promises. You need to do some sorting out yourself about what you expect from this relationship. Why have you put up with Peter's indecision and having to share him with his ex- or almost ex-wife?

JOAN   He has to decide very soon.

THERAPIST   The other issue here that must be clarified is with you, Peter—your relationship to Joan and Cathy. On the surface, it appears as though you are torn between two women, who both want you. However, I think it is more than that. I think you are searching for a warm, loving, nurturing relationship where you feel filled with the goodness that comes from feeling loved. You don't seem to get what you need from either, so you go back and forth, torn between the two, constantly disappointed.

PETER   (nodding and saying quietly) That's exactly how I feel.

THERAPIST   It may be that you do need to sort this out in therapy. Even though you feel that you should be able to figure out and handle your own problems, there are some things that you are too immersed in to be able to sort out by yourself. Neither Joan nor Cathy can help, because they have their own emotional feelings about it.

PETER   Maybe I should see a therapist for a few sessions.

THERAPIST   I think that might be a good idea.

Peter's fear of contact gave important information about how to proceed. He came in as an observer. He didn't respond until I commented on his underlying need. Although I had my own judgment about the issues that Joan and Peter were deliberating about, I knew that it was necessary to focus on what it must feel like for each of them. They were basing their decision-making process on an unusual set of values and beliefs, and their difficulties may or may not have been related to the appropriateness or morality of Peter's relationship to Joan and Cathy. Each of them needed to make a decision that was important to their future.

Joan and Peter did not marry. Peter returned to Chicago and reunited with his wife. Cathy's health problems, if they truly existed, no longer seemed to be an issue. Peter's dilemma of whether to marry Joan or return to his wife was only the tip of the iceberg. He had many underlying issues of vulnerability, neediness, and anger at the failure of the women in his life to meet these needs. Beyond his good looks, charming façade, and his apparent ability to fall passionately in love, Peter felt empty and depressed much of the time. He called me to ask if I could refer him to a therapist near his new home.

Joan married a man 25 years her senior who also worked for the firm and who had long been interested in her. She said they were friends but she had never been attracted to him. But she wanted this baby "more than anything," she said, and religious and family pressure said that marriage was a prerequisite to motherhood. We continued to work together for several months. Joan recognized that her conflicting wish for and fear of intimacy was caused by her early experience with a very self-centered, narcissistically preoccupied mother and a cold distant father. Her major concern in treatment was to assure that she did not do the same thing to her child.

Many people, like Joan and Peter, come into therapy with what they perceive as their reality issues, but upon deeper investigation discover that the precipitating factors are based on unresolved security, loving and bonding needs and anxieties from the past.

Paul and Laura

Paul and Laura had been married 13 years when Paul called for a consultation. Despite the fact that they had had a very good marriage, he said, their relationship had become very tense. Laura was an actress and comedian. In the past she had had a very successful career, but now she was hardly working. Because she had become increasingly depressed about their inability to conceive, he suggested therapy. We had many discussions together about their frustrating attempts at in vitro fertilization, and how it made them feel nonsexual and degraded. They talked of how the baby issue had taken over their lives. Laura spoke of feeling very depressed lately, as every month her menstrual period brought her new disappointment.

In the course of two months of therapy a new option had come up. They had considered a private adoption and were informed that there was a baby they could have. Paul was somewhat reluctant. He considered surrogate parenting a better alternative. He admitted that he really preferred a baby that came from his genes. But after he and Laura discussed it, and she pointed out that this would be their first child and there were many options for future children, including surrogate parenting and the possibility that she would become pregnant, Paul became enthusiastic about the adoption. The week they got the baby they were very happy. They came in for a final session with their infant daughter, Jennifer. A year later, on Jennifer's first birthday, I received a note from them with a picture of a beautiful baby girl.

Shortly afterward Laura called for an appointment. She and Paul were having some trouble communicating, she said, and they seemed to get mad at each other a lot. It was no crisis, she added, but they would like to come in to see me for a few sessions. Now, without a predominant crisis to resolve, many underlying issues arose. In Paul's description of his family history he emerged as the least damaged of three children of an alcoholic, physically abusive father and an intimidated, battered mother. He didn't get beatings as the others did because he learned to talk fast and to run fast. He kept his emotions under check because he knew what damage uncontrolled anger could do.

Laura became increasingly depressed and discouraged that Paul could neither listen to her attempts to share her inner states of mind nor comfort her as he had in the past. Her history revealed a less traumatic childhood. Her mother was depressed and distant, but seemed to come to life in response to Laura's exuberance and sense of humor. Laura learned to entertain very early. By acting the comic, she maintained her position as the family favorite, but at a cost of denying the emergence of a self of her own. She became what her family expected her to be—always happy, friendly, and successful; never showing her sadness, fears or anxieties. No one knew her because she hardly knew herself. Her achievement in the role of "happymaker" compensated for the inner emptiness and depression that she kept in check.

That worked as long as she achieved, but when she stopped getting offers of new roles, and when she was turned down after reading for parts, the depression surged, and demands for attention from Paul increased. She felt rejected and abandoned when he did not respond and was increasingly angry and hurt. He had a great deal of experience in how to avoid anger; he withdrew physically and emotionally. They began by presenting a problem related to the sharing of responsibility of parenting. An added issue, they said, was a lack of communication. The underlying narcissistic issues emerged within a short time.

LAURA We don't talk to each other much anymore. When you're home you are tired or you are doing your work.

PAUL I know—and sometimes I don't feel like talking. I'm feeling upset a lot.

LAURA I think it has been difficult since Jennifer came into our lives. She's been a difficult baby. She's up a lot at night and I need help. It makes us both tense.

PAUL The problem is, I work very hard all day. When I have to get up during the night it's hard to go back to sleep. I go to work bleary-eyed, and it affects my work all day. I don't think that you should expect me to get up with Jennifer at night.

LAURA But you are a parent and parenting is a fifty-fifty proposition. It's important for Jennifer to know both of us are there for her.

PAUL But I am there. I am home every evening. She is awake when I come home and I spend time with her until she goes to sleep. I don't mind taking care of her.

LAURA (Nodding) That's true. You do spend time with her. But I need help at night when she wakes up.

PAUL It's this middle of the night business that makes me so angry. You insist on doing it your way, and you want me to do it your way too.

THERAPIST If I am hearing you both correctly, Laura insists that you share childcare equally because Jennifer needs input from both of you. And Paul is getting increasingly angry about these expectations. It sounds as though this has a lot to do with why you are not communicating well. You may have very different ideas about marriage and childcare.

PAUL I may be a chauvinist, but I cannot help the way I think. I guess I am old-fashioned. I work very hard all day and I earn a lot of money doing it. I arranged it so Laura is one-half owner of our corporation. So she gets a very nice income whether she works or not. When I talk about it she says, "What about my career?" She gave up her theatrical agent, but she still gets calls. Yet she never gets a job that she wants.

LAURA I guess I am waiting for that perfect offer.

PAUL She really doesn't take it that seriously. That bothers me, too.

LAURA The truth is, when I'm out looking for work, I think about being home with Jennifer. When I'm home all day with Jennifer, I think about being out working. I just can't get to a place that feels good.

PAUL The problem is I'm not feeling so good either. You can go to sleep in the afternoon. If I miss my sleep, I still have to go into the office and perform well. I'm a writer, and I work with others. I can't say that I'm tired and want to take a nap. I think to myself, I'm working, I'm bringing in the money that gives us a nice life. You have a housekeeper eight hours a day. (silence for a moment) I guess I'm old-fashioned, but it doesn't feel fair. I feel as though you don't appreciate what I do for us. Sometimes I think about cutting off the checks that you get. Then you might notice what I do for us.

THERAPIST It sounds as though you are angry because Laura seems to get it all, and you end up with all of the work. Laura, I'm sure it seems very different from your viewpoint.

LAURA I love Jennifer, but she is a difficult baby to raise. She was colicky for months and even now is restless a lot. I love to be with her. I just want Paul to spell me sometimes.

PAUL We wouldn't have had as much of a problem if you had listened to me.

THERAPIST What do you mean?

PAUL I read that it's best to let her cry it out and she would then go to sleep. But Laura refused to do that until a couple of weeks ago, when I insisted that we let her cry it out. It is hard for us when the baby is restless and crying. Jennifer cried a lot the first few nights, but now she sleeps through the night.

LAURA I know, I just couldn't stand her crying. It kills me to hear her hurting.

THERAPIST We've spent quite a lot of time today talking about how you handle the problem of Jennifer keeping you up at night. But it sounds as though that is no longer the issue. She's sleeping at night now. The real problems may be how difficult it was for you to resolve it. The fact that you still have very different views on what your roles are in this marriage. And because the way you have tried to resolve things hasn't been very satisfying, there is a lot of frustration and anger that you don't know what to do with. So you don't communicate much of anything. Let's see if we can figure out a little more of this together.

Paul, you sound as though you feel unappreciated for what you bring into the family, as though Laura expects you to do all of what you consider the man's job of supporting the household and then half of her job. So you get angry. But instead of arguing, you withdraw. Then Laura feels alone. she wants you to communicate love, not anger. But you aren't feeling a lot of warmth and loving with this problem hanging over you.

PAUL   That's exactly how I feel. I love Laura and I appreciate all she helped me to do when I was just starting our in this business. She worked a lot then. But now she doesn't seem to want to do anything. She goes for casting calls and interviews. But it's always with the same people. She just socializes all day while the babysitter is with Jennifer.

THERAPIST   As I try to sort this out, something isn't feeling quite right. Laura, you seemed to agree that Paul is with the baby when he gets home. I don't hear you complain that Paul is not a caring father. I also don't see you reacting very much when Paul says how angry he is about your role in the relationship. I'm sure that you are reacting inside though.

LAURA   I don't know what to do. I know I need help with Jennifer sometimes. It makes me too upset when she cries.

THERAPIST   What happens if Paul doesn't help you when you need it?

PAUL   (answering) That's part of what upsets me. She would get up at night if I wouldn't do it. But she would stomp around. And she was rough when she picked up Jennifer. That upset me a lot.

THERAPIST   I wonder about something, Laura. You came in talking about the problem as though it was about sharing childcare. I wonder if there's more to it. I wonder if you are afraid to be with Jennifer sometimes, if you're afraid you can't handle her when she's crying and upset. Maybe that's what you mean when you say that you need Paul to spell you. Maybe you want him to save you from something that feels overwhelming.

LAURA   I love Jennifer. I love to be with her.

PAUL   You are a wonderful mother when everything is perfect. You love being with her when she is happy. And you are a joy to watch when the two of you are playing. But everything has to be perfect.

LAURA You know me. I like to be happy. I like everyone to feel good.

THERAPIST I'm remembering when we worked together a year ago. You were feeling pretty unhappy and depressed. Adopting Jennifer pushed all of those feelings away, at least for a time. But maybe part of what you do for a living is keeping everyone cheered up, including you. Maybe there is a well of unhappiness deep inside. (I could see from the facial muscles and the quiver in her lips that she not only felt what I was describing, but was waiting for an opportunity, or perhaps permission, to cry.) Maybe you have been afraid of your own depression, or your own anger. It might scare you to see it come out when you're upset with Jennifer.

LAURA (At this point tears welled up in Laura's eyes and she looked very small. Paul reached over and put his arms around her. Laura wept for several minutes, as no one said anything.)

THERAPIST Our time is almost up. I want you to know that a lot of people are frightened of what their inside emotions are. Emotions come out in strange ways because to experience them directly hurts too much. It's pretty clear that the problem is not who gets up at night, since you came to see me after Jennifer started sleeping through the night. That gives us a chance to work together on the other things — all of the feelings and emotions that are floating around between you.

LAURA We'll do whatever we have to. I want our marriage to be like it used to.

PAUL I want us to be happy and you to be okay.

THERAPIST This time we may need more sessions than before because we are talking at another level. We can take the time to slowly look at whatever is happening inside of each of you, and how it affects the relationship between you and between both of you and Jennifer.

Laura and Paul had a history of many years of nurturing each other's vulnerable, needy selves. They had been excellent caretakers for each other until the issue of a baby arose. Jennifer's intense affectivity, which was so upsetting to Laura and caused such a problem in the relationship, might have been due to a number of things, not the least of which was the tension in the household that began even before she was adopted. Jennifer was not able to serve the needed function of warding off Laura's sadness and depression. What Laura feared were her inner emotions and the possibility that they would emerge and overwhelm her. She needed someone there to protect her. As she began to work through her feelings, Paul was surprised at how much his memory clicked into having many of the same early feelings as Laura did. As they touched upon areas of narcissistic vulnerability, each came to understand the reasons for the heretofore confusing reactions of the other. Previously they had little to say to each other because what they were feeling raised fears that exposure would result in the destruction of the relationship. The open sharing of hurts and anger reactions was the beginning of renewed ability to connect emotionally.

For over 20 years I have been trying to understand why some couples break up while others take the same issues in stride. I have heard people in therapy say with certainty that their mates are "crazy" or "acting irrationally." What they mean by this is that the reactions of their mates do not make sense to them. Just as the "unreasonable patient" (Giovacchini, 1987) can be understood if the therapist's listening perspective is trained to hear the intrinsic message, the "illogical" behavior of a mate makes sense when one tunes into the underlying messages being communicated.

CHAPTER 7

Acting-out as an Expression of Narcissistic Vulnerability

As we have seen in Chapter 6, presenting problems frequently stem from underlying narcissistic vulnerability. This chapter will continue that discussion with a consideration of the surface problems—acting-out—which betray underlying pathology. Marital partners may not even be aware that they are subject to excessive vulnerability. Instead, one or both spouses act out through rages, affairs, or addictions—to anything from alcohol to shopping. Sometimes a child who has been drawn into a collusive pattern becomes depressed or engages in delinquent acts, unconsciously maintaining the painful family equilibrium. The basis of the problem remains the same. Partners, preoccupied with their vulnerabilities, live in terror (Lansky, 1981) and must defend their fragile selves. Acting-out behavior reduces the experience of overwhelming stress, anxiety, or terror.

When internal experiences become more than the person's protective barriers or habitual defenses can handle, the result may be a somatic acting-in or behavioral acting-out. The former may cause tension and stress that comes out in the body, such as difficulty in speech or bodily functions, or physical illness. How such "acting-in" is affected by individual psychological and somatic problems is described extremely well in McDougall's *Theaters of the Mind* and *Theaters of the Body*. When illness is utilized for secondary gain in a relationship, it is, in a sense, acting-out behavior.

In acting-out behavior, one deceives not only one's partner but also oneself. Facing the pain of unmet narcissistic needs must be avoided at all costs. "I am under so much stress from my new job that my stomach is upset all of the time and I am too exhausted to do my share of the work at home." "My job is important for the welfare of our family." . . . "If you loved me you would understand." "If you don't do what I want, you are not interested in my welfare . . . then I have a right to be very angry at you." "If you continue to not understand my needs, then I have a right to seek understanding from someone else." Such are the internal explanations for whatever behavior follows.

AFFAIRS

A common presenting problem bringing couples into marital therapy is the extramarital affair. However, while many people blame affairs for the breakup of their marriage, affairs do not happen in a vacuum. They are symptoms of underlying problems or attempts to deny such problems. An affair is an emotionally charged series of events among husband, wife, and a third party enlisted to complete the triangle. Affairs have a variety of causes, but for the most part they are representations of underlying narcissistic needs. An affair may function as a distance regulator, as an instrument of revenge, as the expression of a need for an affirming other, as a way to convince oneself of one's attractiveness, sexual potency or lovableness, or as the expression of a desire to play.

Like other aspects of relationships, affairs occur on several levels at the same time. On the first level there is the presenting problem, sometimes emerging when the affair is discovered by the mate. Figure 7.1 gives some examples of the surface and underlying layers of an affair.

The decision to become involved in an affair is a self-focused indulgence. A neurotic mechanism may allow one to rationalize the affair as making things better for the marriage. "It has added variety to my responses to my husband," said one woman. "What she doesn't know won't hurt her," explained a man who was turning 50 and sought reassurance that he was still attractive to women. Affairs sometimes are attempts at aggrandizement of an impoverished self. "I am just a very sexual person and need lots of variety," said a man who was compulsively involved in repeated sexual conquests. When narcissistic defenses are in operation, the affair often serves the purpose of retaliation and triumph over another. "She doesn't respond as I need. Well, there are lots of other women who will." "I need someone to hold me and tell me that I am loved. He loves only his work, so I am entitled to find pleasure elsewhere."

Falling in love is a delightful experience of total narcissistic fulfillment. The cooperative, even eager merging of boundaries provides an unsurpassed experience of wholeness and uniqueness. For the psychologically

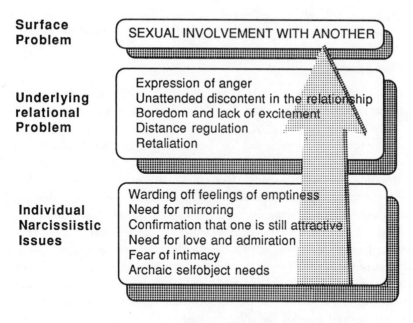

FIGURE 7.1
Issues Underlying Acting-Out Behavior

healthy individual it is a supremely pleasurable experience. For the narcissisticly fragile self whose whole being feels impermanent, falling in love may be an unaccustomed experience of complete wholeness. If the feeling of falling in love is combined with a fear that one's self-boundaries may dissolve and anxiety about being "swallowed up" by another, what occurs is a series of relationships that last only until the other asks, "Where is this relationship going?" "When do my needs get met?" "Why do you never seem to be there for me?" At that point there is a fear of being trapped and the affair is terminated. The explanation is often that "my wife (and/or my children) need me. . . . I cannot leave them." The wife and children protect the narcissist from being caught in a relationship that is becoming too intimate. At the same time, the affair is a protection against the danger of the marriage being too intimate. Affairs thus serve many purposes in maintaining a fragile self.

The affair may be discovered accidentally, may be flaunted in order to get a reaction, or may become public, thus forcing the mate to acknowledge what was known but denied for a long time. Despite the attendant guilt, an affair often results in the temporary enhancement of the person's feelings of attractiveness and acceptance. An outside relationship also changes the power positions and interactional contract of the partners.

Shauna and Sam

Shauna informed her husband, Sam, that she was leaving him for the contractor who had been working on their home. His reaction was to fight to save the marriage. For the first time in years he put aside his work and became totally involved in her life. Remembering how much in love they had been, he was not about to let another man win her away. Her affair, at that point, reactivated a dying relationship. They worked together in therapy for several months. Sam described his initial feeling of unbelievable good luck to have won Shauna over her many other suitors. She came from a wealthy family, and he was determined to outsucceed her father. He did succeed in an international business, calling Europe at 6 a.m. and the Orient at midnight. If they could only amass enough money, they could live as he had always promised they would. He hardly noticed her involvement with her lover, despite the many signals that she purposely left. Only when she told him of the affair and her decision to leave him did he recognize that they had a problem.

When an affair is uncovered, if the couple can talk about it the marriage may survive and may even grow from the experience, as Sam and Shauna's marriage did. By the time an affair begins, however, the relationship is already in trouble. Below the surface of the affair there are generally a great many relational issues.

Hank and Patricia

Hank fought for years with his wife about how unsatisfying their sex life was. What he found pleasurable, Patricia did not enjoy. What she wanted was extended foreplay followed by unhurried intercourse that would enable her to achieve orgasm. She read the many books on sexuality and knew that there must be more than she was feeling with Hank. But when she tried to talk to him about it, he became very uncomfortable and blamed her for their sexual problems. She recognized that their inability to discuss and resolve their problems was specific to this relationship, because she had no difficulty being open and honest with others. But working out anything with Hank had become increasingly difficult and she almost gave up trying.

She declined Hank's suggestion that they try different sexual activities and positions that might be more satisfying. If he won't talk, she won't play.

She no longer cared if they resolved the sexual issue, she told him. The problem was his premature ejaculation, and she was not willing to accept responsibility for this. Increasingly he was impotent on the occasions when Patricia agreed to sexual relations. From Hank's point of view, oral sex, which he considered normal, she thought of as animalistic and dirty. She insisted on her terms and her "healthy" way of behaving sexually.

He threatened that he would go elsewhere to meet his sexual needs. Ultimately he did. He immersed himself in an affair which reassured him and confirmed his potency. It was not a very clandestine affair, as he dropped hints at varying times, and Patricia soon found out about it. Her response was a threat to divorce him and take the children back to the city where her parents lived. It was at this point that they sought therapy. Their unsatisfying relationship was being acted out through the sexual impasse and the affair. Their many other issues related to internal conflict, feelings of shame and guilt, and need for distance regulation emerged later.

Sexuality is generally only a small part of what is wrong in a marriage. Women who become involved in an affair often have a history of complaints that their husband is not there for them emotionally. They want more touching, more nonsexual holding, more talk about the relationship. They want to know that they are loved. Men often have a very different view of how to show love. "I married you, didn't I?" has a very different meaning for a man than for a woman. He is saying, "I made a commitment to you." The wife hears, "Don't act so childishly. I shouldn't have to be bothered constantly reassuring you of my love." The fantasy of most women who become involved in extramarital affairs is that there will be someone to talk to, someone who understands them, someone who makes them feel fulfilled.

The generally secretive nature of affairs makes it almost impossible to know the exact percentages of marriages in which one or both partners have been involved in sexual relationships outside of marriage. Sexual researchers have suggested that 45–55% of wives and 50–65% of husbands are, at some point in marriage, involved in outside affairs (Nass, Libby, and Fisher, 1981). The result of the affair can range from the destruction of the marriage to the reestablishment of the commitment on a new basis.

ADDICTIONS

Kevin and Roseanne

Many times when I see couples who are having difficulties, one or both are misusing food, alcohol, or drugs. For instance, Kevin, who was very disappointed in his relationships, treated his pain with alcohol. Throughout his life Kevin tried to make everyone happy. As a child he denied his parents' messages that they were unhappy because he feared the breakup of his family. He thought that if he was always cheerful and a "big boy" they would stay together. He failed. His fantasy of marriage was that he would create the perfect family where everyone would be happy. He ignored his wife's messages of unhappiness until she became so dissatisfied with what she called his "immature behavior" that she refused to even talk to him. She told him that she would stay with him because of the children, but would not go with him to therapy because it was hopeless. He felt totally alone. There was no one to hold him, to love him, to make love to. "I came close to having an affair," he said, "but knew in my heart that wasn't the answer. It would endanger the marriage, and I might lose my children." He entered individual treatment with the stated goal of improving the relationship.

One day he talked about having a second and then a third drink when he arrived home from work. He mentioned going for lunch to a local bar. "It's like *Cheers*," he said, "a place where they know me and I feel welcome." One day he said, "I feel guilty when I tell you about taking a few drinks. I wonder why. I don't have a drinking problem." I responded that he had a reason for bringing it up and had hinted at misusing alcohol on several occasions and mused, "I wonder if the drinking fills the emptiness that you feel when Roseanne keeps you at such an emotional distance." As we examined his drinking pattern he recognized how much he drank when he was alone. Alcohol served the safe, consistent nurturing needs that he so desperately sought. He recognized that he was on the way to having a drinking problem. Kevin, who had always denied anything painful, began to talk about his needy, demanding self. He recognized how his behavior had always kept him in the position of needing to be cared for. The surface level of acting-out gave way to an internal world of self needs and fears.

Another young man, newly married and already talking about divorce, came in with his bride of five months. "He never leaves his computer," she complained. "He comes home from work, eats dinner quickly, and goes to his IBM. It's like he is having a love affair. I can't get in at all. When I interrupt, he becomes enraged." She left him shortly afterward.

Computers have become a serious addiction for some people, enhancing fragile self-images. For those who feel confused, unloved, and anxious, the computer is a friend who fills many needs. The clear structure of the computer leaves them in total control. Do it right and all things are possible. For some the computer is a transitional object from childhood to the world of adults; for others it has become an addiction, a provider of functions that allow withdrawal from the world. It demands nothing and always responds when it is turned on, the perfect object for narcissistic relatedness. But for the most part computer addicts have few satisfying personal relationships, since under stress they withdraw into a world that responds as needed. The language of psychotherapy often is experienced as quite alien to computer addicts, who value logic and function over emotion and feeling. Suggestions that they examine underlying aspects of the self, which cannot be counted and measured, are met with resistance.

An addiction that is seldom identified as such is shopping. There are some people who spend their days in shopping malls because they only feel good when they are buying something. In therapy it is often the husband who complains that his wife is ruining him with her charge cards. In one situation there were no marital complaints until the husband's business faltered and almost went bankrupt. The wife agreed that she was a compulsive shopper and wondered how to stop. She hoped there was a quick cure because she would prefer to spend her money on clothes rather than therapy. Later she acknowledged that she continued in therapy only because they had an insurance policy that covered it. During the time that we worked together in marital therapy, her husband came to see how obsessed she had become with buying. She loved bargains because they proved that the time she spent was valuable. She loved having new dresses and getting compliments on them. She loved the feeling of fullness that she experienced when she was able to buy something that she wanted.

Charles and Andrea

Another couple, Charles and Andrea, did not have financial problems. She had always loved to shop, but as a single woman could only charge so much before her credit stopped. Once she and Charles married, however, there was a seemingly endless supply of money. They spent their time looking for ways to consume. They flew first class from Los Angeles to New York merely to have dinner or see a show. They went on unusual and very expensive vacations. Charles, who had made a fortune in real estate, could not get over the fact that he was wealthy.

One day Charles attempted suicide. He went into analysis, where he described a lifetime of feeling depressed. Only when he was doing, achieving, moving at a very fast pace, spending, acquiring, and making more money had he been able to tolerate the feeling that he had no right to exist at all. He needed to stop all his activities in order to evaluate himself and his life. His wife, supportive and wishing to help, did not know how to change her own pattern of spending. They entered marital therapy while he continued to work on his own inner issues.

Slowly Charles learned to endure long periods of depression without running from the anxieties that came upon him. He moved to further understanding of his anger and disappointment that his own parents never seemed to draw him toward vitality and life. He recognized his need to stimulate himself because no one in his experience did it for him. When his wife asked where she fit in, he explained that his goal was to stimulate and entertain all of the people around him. That was his childhood role, he realized, with his depressed mother and his distant and withdrawn father. Charles spent six years in analysis tracing the threads of his early life interactions. Charles and Andrea together worked in marital therapy for close to five years. Although they continued to live well, the spending addiction that had become a refuge from major depression was no longer an issue.

Drug addictions are the most difficult to break and, along with alcoholism, the most destructive to relationships. Such addictions are not only psychological but also physical. Drugs give the feeling of omnipotence, of perfection, of driving away the destructive or empty core self. The sexual response may feel enhanced, although it actually decreases. Grandiosity and omnipotence prevail while the drug is in effect. Relationships are subordinated to the search for new supplies, while whatever underlying rage reactions exist are given free reign.

BLAMING, ATTACKING AND RAGE REACTIONS

In healthy marriages, conflict remains rooted in a specific situation and, to a certain extent, in the current messages of society. The spouses ask for what they want or can be taught to ask in therapy. In narcissistic relationships with severe pathology, however, attack and withdrawal are common patterns. In attacking marriages, anger always seems to be present. One seemingly small issue after another is used to justify the expression of infantile rage. Disagreements become opportunities for vengeful assault. Harmony in such an attacking relationship is maintained only so long as perfect mirroring responses are undisturbed. Such marriages can continue for years in superficial equilibrium unless overwhelming stress undermines their fragile foundations. While each partner functions well in the outside world, and the marriage even seems quite comfortable to others who observe it from the outside, rage wells up in response to lapses in approving or affirming responses. The experience of being failed and of psychic injury is much greater than the partner or an outside observer can fathom.

In relationships where splitting and projective identification are the primary defenses, partners put into each other the hate-filled images that are too awful to acknowledge in themselves. Hostile, dependent relationships between people who can neither live with nor without each other are filled with translocated and "dumped out" feelings. Such relationships are difficult to treat in marital therapy because each mate has important psychological reasons to maintain the relationship for individual internal (although pathological) stability.

Coming to terms with the split between good and bad enables the person to accept and tolerate ambivalence. It is not until the loving and hating elements of self and other coalesce, permitting ambiguity, that the defense of splitting can be given up. Only in this way can feelings of anger be held without fear that they will destroy the other or the self. Then it is possible to be angry at the temporary frustration of one's desires without danger and without evoking reactions of narcissistic rage.

All people, including "normal" neurotics, carry within them certain pockets of psychosis (S. Klein, 1981; Tustin, 1987) and may experience episodes during which the observing ego is lost. Some rationalize the affect that expands to an explosion, blaming the rage on the person or object nearest to them. Since the other is the cause, whatever happens is exactly what they deserve. "I expect you to read my mind and think as I do" is the unspoken command of the narcissist who needs mirroring. There is a wish that the partner will always be properly responsive. When the partner fails, a rage wells up within that can be frightening to both.

Ed and Sandra

Ed went to see a therapist with his dilemma. He loved his wife, Sandra, but sometimes when he got angry at her he "lost it." If she forgot to remind him of something he was supposed to do, or if she was late coming home from work, his upset feelings turned explosive. He tried to control his temper, but when those events happened he had no control. When it was over he would not discuss it. He just wanted to forget it—to pretend it had not happened.

One evening Ed became enraged because there was no beer in the refrigerator. Although he and Sandra were at the market together, he did not remember to buy beer, nor did she. When they returned home, he was angry that she did not care for him enough to remember. He began throwing things and broke a vase that they both loved. Later he could not explain why he became furious or why he did so with increasing frequency. Fearing loss of control and loss of his wife, he responded to her suggestion and sought therapy. However, when he suggested that Sandra join him for conjoint sessions, she declined, and he terminated. Sandra, believing that the problem rested entirely in Ed, was not interested in treatment. "If you change, we will be fine," she insisted with great conviction.

Sandra, vulnerable herself and easily wounded, did not recognize her part in the problems of the relationship. She constructed a shell to protect herself and started to withdraw, leaving Ed to experience old feelings of abandonment. She was reluctant to come out of this shell with him because she never knew just when he might "explode." The reciprocity of his abuse when feelings of narcissistic rage emerged and her need to maintain a protective shell to avoid shattering attacks resulted in each avoiding closeness with the other.

The pattern became fixed, a script for a marriage in which partners cannot live with or without each other. Instead they alternated between periods of anxious calm and series of intolerable arguments. Sandra threatened to leave, or Ed told her to do so on numerous occasions. Each, at times, considered departing permanently. Occasionally, after a flare-up, one or the other actually did leave, but the separations were short-lived. Before the day was over, either Sandra or Ed was on the telephone, imploring the other to make up. So they have continued, not wanting the emptiness that floods them when they are alone, not able to avoid the intense pain of living together. They cherish the tranquility of the calm periods, hoping that the latest blowup was the last one.

Unfortunately, it is in such relationships that escalating rage may recur and begin to be acted out in physical as well as emotional attacks, something that is more frequent than is generally known or admitted. We assume that intelligent, sophisticated people do not lose control and hit each other. That is not what I hear in my office. At first I hear a single remark, a mention of some extreme provocation. "It was 2 a.m. and she hadn't come home. I went to her girlfriend's house and they were both drunk. I tried to get her to come home, but she wanted to stay. So I hit her—it was just a little slap." Then, as we discuss it, I hear more details about the increasingly violent fights that they had been ashamed to discuss. Little issues expand into huge battles. Battles escalate into someone pushing or throwing something. For instance, Sy and Lori, both cocaine users, broke china, chairs, tables, walls, and doors. She threw all of his clothes in the swimming pool, and he retaliated by pushing her car into the pool. If such behavior is not stopped instantly, the message is that the inner control of rage can be released with impunity. Each time it occurs, the abusing partner or both abusing partners find it that much easier to allow anger to turn into physical violence. Often, once such abuse takes hold in a relationship it continues until a physical separation stops it.

Walter and Marge

Walter, a successful screenwriter, describes a welling up of rage as "a ball of fire—like a tight fist in my solar plexus." He adds, "A membrane surrounds this ball of fury; the membrane is fear." The more frightened he becomes, Walter explains, the tighter the membrane shrinks and the more he tries to withdraw from the pain. When the terror becomes unbearable, the membrane breaks and the fury is released. Once released, the rage turns "icy cold," uncaring of consequence, destructive of anything in its path. "This state is not me," he says. "When Marge starts picking on me, I can feel it coming. I feel the breaking point coming, and sometimes try to get her to stop or get away." Walter believes that there is something "crazy" welling up within him. He feels it often: When he is cut off by a car on the freeway he sometimes chases after the car to cut the other driver off. When he is thwarted at work he feels the churning inside, the membrane containing the rage stretching to near the breaking point. At work he knows he must not lose control. He keeps the lid on and waits until it passes, until the fury and the fear subside. At home he can release it.

Then he says that if Marge would just stop doing things that upset him he would not explode at her like that. She should understand. He works hard to support her and the kids. He has enough aggravation at work. Why does she keep doing things that "blow him out of his mind"? he asks. Then he blames her—it is not him. Why does she not understand and just stop doing things to make him so mad?

As soon as he has vented his fury on Marge, he is rid of it. He becomes calm. Since it is not really he, and it is her fault anyway, he is over it quickly. He barely remembers that he has just assaulted Marge with a huge blast of intolerable fury. Of course he is correct in believing that she is constantly furious with him. She has become increasingly enraged but hides her feelings out of fear. She waits for the moments when it will be over.

For hours or days he is free of the rage and there is peace. Both hope it is finished—that it will never happen again. But it will. As long as he believes that it is Marge's failure to respond properly to his needs that cause his rages, he will feel entitled to evacuate his feelings into her when they become intolerable. As long as Marge accepts what he projects into her, it will continue. Each time the rage wells up it surprises her. When it is gone she hopes it is gone forever.

Marge was abused as a child, so she is repeating a past experience. She does not know what it is she is doing that provokes Walter's behavior. She does not consciously accept his rationalization that it is her fault. Yet she doesn't believe that she has any alternative. She is terrified by his rages but chooses to be married to him because of the status, the social position, and the peaceful periods between the rages. He is talented, extremely smart, interested in many of the things that she loves. When their marriage is good, it is very good.

The alternative, she believes, is to be alone. So she does nothing. Sometimes she has suggested that he go into therapy. He says that nothing is wrong with him. She has suggested marital counseling; he refuses. He is not hurting as long as he can relieve himself of his anger by putting it onto her.

This was their pattern for many years. Then Marge began to change. As her own anger accumulated, she began to have headaches, backaches, and stomachaches. She had wanted to have a baby but was glad that she had not yet been able to conceive. One day she came to the realization that the marriage was making her sick. She decided to get a divorce. She was firm in her decision and moved into an apartment that they owned near the beach.

Walter was shocked. He remembered only the good things they had had together, in spite of what he saw as her sometimes provocative actions. Her moving out was just one more piece of incomprehensible behavior. He was surprised at how intolerably empty he felt without her. He did not realize how much he depended on her presence. He suggested that they get therapy. He was even willing to see a therapist himself.

He was fortunate in that she agreed. Sometimes, by the time the partner faces the possibility of having to divorce, the experience of separation is such a great relief that the fluctuations of an erratic relationship can no longer be tolerated. There is a fear of being drawn into another self-destructive experience.

In conjoint therapy Marge learned to understand her role in Walter's rages. She also realized that he became enraged when she disagreed with him, when she failed to read his mind, when she did things that reminded him of her separateness. She stopped taking responsibility for his uncontrolled emotions. She came to recognize that she did not have to act in ways that avoided reminding him that she had a self of her own. If he was unable to contain his own feelings, she had the right to walk away—out of the house or out of his life. She was no longer willing to be a victim. He recognized that he could contain his anger with colleagues at work and with friends; therefore, he could do the same at home. He had not done so because he did not need to.

Once Marge refused to accept his rage, her self-esteem grew and they began the slow process of change. Realizing that she was serious, Walter made a real effort to understand. He recognized a lifelong pattern of needing to have someone nearby and of finding it difficult to maintain a comfortable relationship. He reexamined his anger at his mother for her intrusive demandingness and came to understand how this carried over into adulthood; even now, when he talks with his mother on the telephone he regularly hangs up in anger.

As we saw in Part One, and as Walter and Marge learned, anger and rage are components of narcissistic injury and defense. It is not unusual to see intense anger being suppressed or acted out in relationships between family members. The acting-out of anger through physical violence is sometimes explained with the excuse, "I was provoked," or "She drove me to it," or "I was only trying to stop what was happening." That statement is intended to minimize or mitigate the violence as just something that happens occasionally when they argue. But when anger is acted out in hitting, pushing or beating another person, it tends to reduce the underlying inhibitions. For some people it feels better to act it out, and so the violence increases. It is injurious to both husband and wife to allow the violent acting-out behavior without immediately telling them that it is deleterious to both the marriage and the therapeutic work.

Rage is not reduced by its discharge in action; instead it increases (Gaylin, 1984). It is difficult enough to work with marriages in which there is a split between love and hate, where rageful feelings emerge whenever the partner fails to respond as wished. When feelings are acted out in a physical manner, treatment is unproductive.

The purpose of acting-out is the avoidance of unacceptable affectivity. The critical factor in psychic development is whether frustration or anxiety is avoided or whether the attempt is made to come to terms with it. Effective psychotherapy requires that intense emotions not be discharged but tolerated long enough to understand and modify their effects. The therapist's role with the couple is to make the sessions a place where feelings and fears can be identified and dangerous impulses explored in terms of how they occurred in the past, what brings them up in the present, how they affect the relationship, and how they are contained. This requires a clear understanding of how the therapeutic environment can be made a holding place for hard-to-contain feelings until they can be brought to awareness and communicated in ways other than acting-out. The following chapters will describe how this can be accomplished in conjoint therapy with couples.

CHAPTER 8

Initial Treatment Considerations

When supportive mutuality exists, marital therapy can repair both the system and the mates. Treatment must take into account the pattern of interactions, as well as the health or pathology of the system and the disturbance of each of the individuals involved. Individual pathology is played out in family relationships through patterns of verbal and nonverbal communication.

Effective treatment requires both understanding of how partners attempt to use verbal and nonverbal communication to enhance understanding of aspects of themselves that are unknown to either and awareness of how communication patterns are utilized to protect a vulnerable self from injury. The conduct of marital therapy and conscious and unconscious communication in marriage are the topics of Chapters 9 and 10; here I will focus on how an understanding of psychodynamic factors influences assessment and treatment goals in conjoint therapy.

As we have seen in Part One, marriages are made not in heaven but in the earliest dynamic interactions between parent and child, which are repeatedly reenacted in adult relationships. In well-functioning marriages partners develop an empathic understanding of each other's needs and find ways of demonstrating care and affirmation to each other. As a result they become more tolerant of existing archaic needs, both in their partner and in themselves.

Some couples come into therapy sharing neurotic disorders colored by narcissistic injury; others seek help for manifestations of their individual and collective borderline-narcissistic disorders (Lachkar, 1985; Solomon, 1985). Even marriages of relatively psychologically healthy but unhappily relating individuals may be at risk for narcissistic turmoil, simply because current problems cause mates to feel burdened by a sense of self-esteem that is to some degree compromised and uncertain (Scharff and Scharff, 1987, p. 350). Because of this, the treatment methods described here may be applied with a wide range of couples. They are, however, particularly applicable to those individuals who feel so vulnerable that even small hurts are experienced as exquisitely painful and to those who find that allowing any closeness with others causes the emergence of intolerable affect.

Engaging in marital therapy may, at first, heighten the partners' degree of self-consciousness and shame. The ground feels less solid when one must ask for help on issues as personal as those that arise out of failures in a marriage. For many people, the idea of seeing a therapist to discuss problems with a spouse is extremely anxiety-provoking. Depending on the person's sense of inner cohesiveness, engagement in therapy may produce varying narcissistic defenses.

Rarely do couples begin therapy with the belief or even the wish that the therapist will remain unbiased in the assignment of responsibility for correcting an impaired relationship. The usual fantasy is that the problems of the relationship lie within the mate. If only the therapist had a clear picture of how unfeeling, inconsiderate, or hurtful the other has been, then the therapist would find a way of resolving the current problem – by getting the partner to change. Of course, at another level each partner is aware of the distortions in such an account. Often, at a deeper level lies the opposing fear that some inner emptiness, badness, or unworthiness in oneself is the cause of all the unhappiness.

In most instances, when couples seek therapy to help a relationship, the partners have not been able to adequately provide needed functions for one another. The result is a great deal of unhappiness, and generally a clear presenting symptom in at least one of the partners or in their children. Ultimately, the frustration of narcissistic expectations causes what appears to be a breakdown of communication. Attempts to get the partners to talk directly to each other can prolong a mutually collusive and destructive process. Consequently, a different communicative approach is necessary with the narcissistically vulnerable who are building a reparative relationship.

Even two people whose individual sense of self is less than optimal may assume complementary roles for each other. If there is a mutuality of needs and strengths that help them to supply needed functions for each other, individuals with extreme narcissistic vulnerabilities may experience a reduction of chronic anxiety and even begin to interact with others outside the relationship in new ways. Thus, the intensity of individual clinical symptoms may decrease. On the other hand, when mates' world views do not coincide in mutually supportive ways, the interaction can become increasingly painful. Treatment of a dysfunctional relationship demands, therefore, an intensive exploration of both partners' needs, of their prevailing inability to communicate and satisfy those needs, and of the resulting emotional and affective chaos that emerges in times of stressful interaction.

For example, when there is a preexisting vulnerability to narcissistic injury, intensive emotional exploration may cause an explosive reaction. Each partner has been hurt and is prepared to defend against any blow to an already damaged self. Each wishes for unconditional acceptance and affirmation. Each looks to the other to make the marriage into the safe haven that was missing in earlier life. In the context of a fragmenting adult relationship, there is a tendency to replay old traumas, fears, disappointments, and defense patterns. Disagreements serve as reminders of old unmet needs and unmended failures. This results in the reemergence of internal experiences from early family life, with all of the attendant blame, shame and rage. The lack of emotional warmth that characterizes a relationship affected by narcissistic vulnerability has as its counterpart excessive expectations that neither partner is capable of fulfilling for the other.

TREATMENT GOALS

A long-term goal of conjoint therapy is the *reshaping of the inner representations* partners have of each other. This occurs when interventions shift the nature of the couple's interactions, disconfirming images they have of each other as unloving, ungiving, or malevolent. At this stage they are helped as mates to reveal deeper levels of feeling, as each is assured that the other can hear and accept. Still later it is possible for the mates to engage in individual treatment to deal with the problems that first came out in marital interactions. Nevertheless, after a period of conjoint marital therapy, partners are often able to relate to each other in ways that are less destructive to the marriage, despite continuing individual personal problems.

A second goal is to *help partners become aware of some of the emotions that lie below the surface* of their carefully scripted fights over things that they "know." For example, each may be aware of being upset and troubled in the relationship, without understanding the true nature of what is so troubling. Recognition of the cause of the despair brings them too close to emotions that are unacceptably shameful, guilt-producing, or terrifying.

During this process, the challenge in conjoint therapy sessions is to maintain an equidistant, even-handed position that includes responsiveness to the underlying internal experience of both partners, so that neither is identified as the cause of the problem or the more disturbed one. Each spouse must feel safe enough to present his or her experience of the relationship and feel heard at least by the therapist and, as soon as possible, by the partner.

Insight into one's own or a mate's early dynamics does not necessarily result in change. In fact, it may further damage an already deteriorating relationship. For example, whenever Earl and Peggy fought, he alluded to the unhappy relationship her parents had, as well as to her own frustrating relationship with her father. "You are just treating me like your mother treated your father," he said, "and I won't stand for it." The communication ended there, even as their voices escalated. "At least my father didn't leave home for days at a time to be with a girlfriend, like yours did." "My parents' problems have nothing to do with your constant nagging." There is no way to resolve such disputes; the partners are not even aware of what sets off the arguments. Despite the recognition that negative feelings toward each other may come from problems initiating in childhood, this couple lacks the specific skills to use that comprehension constructively.

Sometimes the situation is complicated by the fact that recreation of early unresolved problems occurs in intimate relationships, while in the world outside the home the partners relate well to others and function competently. As soon as they get home, they find themselves in impossible situations again. They fight continuously over subjects as insignificant as where to store the dog food, dinner plans, and whether or not to shop at certain markets. While it distresses them that they cannot stop fighting, it seems impossible for them to discuss everyday subjects in a rational manner.

It is extraordinarily difficult for those with split-off affective reactions to hear and accept an interpretation of their relationship difficulties. When problems are pointed out, they are quickly put out of conscious awareness. Thus, it is better to discuss in detail each partner's painful feelings or anxieties before discussing ways they could handle the situation. Insight alone will not resolve marital problems; something must be done to change the underlying structure that is provoking current interactions.

When the process of gaining insight is not experienced as an assault or a potential cause of narcissistic injury, defensive measures will not have to be taken to protect the vulnerable structures of each partner's self. The recognition that, in the therapist's presence, each one is going to be heard and responded to, rather than besieged with blame and guilt-producing responses, is the first step in the curative process of marital treatment.

A third goal of a psychodynamic approach to marital therapy is to *keep anxiety within tolerable limits while helping each individual to reintegrate split-off feelings*. Over time the result of this process is a reshaping of internal representations of self and other, the enhancement of self-esteem, and greater well-being of the relationship.

The significant interventions in marital therapy take place at the intersection at which self and object meet, as diagramed in Figure 8.1. An important goal is the *exploration of how partners use each other to enhance vigor and vitality and to maintain their own self-cohesion*. Where ineffective attempts to exchange important emotional needs within the marital unit underlie dysfunctional relationships, new paths must be developed. When one partner makes overwhelming demands or fails to accept the other's basic need for differentiation of self, the reasons for the specific reactions must be explored. The work of treatment is done in the relational space between husband, wife, and therapist.

Note the similarity between Figure 8.1 and Figure 4.1 (p. 68), a diagram describing intersubjective relatedness in child development. The process is essentially the same in both instances. As the infant becomes increasingly

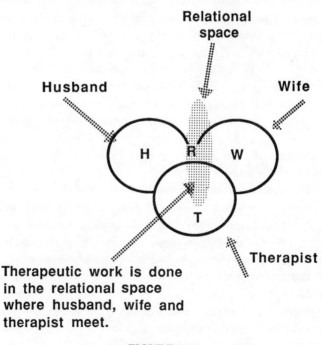

FIGURE 8.1
The Relational Space

aware of the outer environment, the internal action moves from omnipotent self-centeredness to generalized patterns of interactions with others; in the interactional space where self and other overlap and sometimes merge, relationships develop. This relational space is common to the dynamics of both parent-child and patient-therapist interactions. Each provides an arena for growth and change. Therapy is focused on observing and reflecting upon what occurs in the relational space between husband and wife, then between the couple and therapist, and finally between each individual partner and the therapist.

THE FIRST INTERVIEW

The first stage of treatment involves forming an alliance between the couple and therapist in which both partners feel understood. Each spouse must experience safety in sharing not only with the therapist but also with the other. The therapist's demonstration of empathic listening encourages the spouses to try and understand each other. The therapist, in addition, must help each partner to verbalize rather than act out feelings and to identify and give words to feelings that seem too painful to express.

The initial conjoint session is an exploration. The couple and therapist size each other up. Some couples enter into therapy and even idealize the therapist without asking questions about the therapist's training and orientation or about the therapist's attitudes toward marriage and marital problems. Others have more specific expectations of conjoint therapy than they might have of individual treatment; they know that they are seeking someone who treats marital problems.

In the formation of a working alliance, the goal is to enlist the observing ego of each partner in a mutual journey toward a common outcome. The therapist may encounter some dead ends and make some errors in attempting to balance understanding of two sometimes widely divergent points of view. If misunderstandings occur too often, or if one or both of the mates are particularly vulnerable to feelings of being blamed or attacked, the working alliance needed to achieve the goals of treatment might not develop.

Gurman (1977, p. 436) suggests that some people experience an alliance with the therapist although they receive only the therapist's warmth and empathy. Others require interactional insight, such as identification of repetitive patterns of behavior, or genetic insight, such as connecting current patterns to past relationships with parents. Still others seek at least minimal direction for behavior change outside the treatment.

From the moment they come into the consulting room, marriage partners give clues about many aspects of their difficulties and their resources for dealing with problems. As they sit silently or talk together in the waiting room, the therapist can observe their ages, mode of dress, appearance of alertness or depression. What nonverbal and verbal clues do they give as they come into the office? Where do they sit—on a single couch, in separate chairs, across the room from each other?

When I ask my usual beginning question—"Can you tell me why you decided to come in to see me?"—I watch for who responds first. Does one talk for both? Are there any signs of disagreement or nonverbal signs of hurt? I do not ask specific questions about age, occupation, children, and so on, because this information is on a one-page information form new patients are asked to fill out in the waiting room. At this early stage I am more interested in the process of their interaction. Issues around relationships with children, parents and in-laws invariably emerge in the course of discussing current problems. Each partner's history may come up spontaneously during the early discussion or in response to specific questions.

The main task during this initial process is to tap into the other alliance, the transitional space between partners in the marital relationship. In presenting their problem, the spouses will provide clues to the central conflict or to some issue that has disrupted a previously adaptive pattern. These clues are more often than not presented in disguised or derivative messages (Langs, 1976b). It is the task of the therapist to translate these into meaningful messages about needs and fears in the here and now of the current relationship. The therapist becomes aware of the way partners maintain an unspoken contract that links them together. In order to examine recurrent interactional patterns and the role each partner plays (caretaker, frightened child, etc.), the therapist must be able to maintain boundaries separate from the couple and yet at times enter into their boundaries.

While the couple together presents content messages the therapist observes through several modalities, they also present clues about each partner's way of being in a relationship. A great deal of information is provided early in treatment, often more than can be consciously incorporated and used. As the therapist probes aspects of the couple's life together, observation of interactions gives clues to the inner representational world of each of them. Their descriptions of their desires for the marriage and of their current relationship to their children and parents give information about how to proceed. Therapists must also train themselves in the use of their own and others' intense emotions to provide important diagnostic information; this will be discussed in greater detail in Chapter 11 in the section on countertransference as a therapeutic tool.

The tools used to make diagnostic assessments are of several types.

There are observations of the mates' transference reactions toward each other and toward the therapist; there are the therapist's countertransference reactions not only toward the individuals involved but also toward the couple as a unit. Information about the family history and sociocultural background of each partner constitutes important data. Taking a careful history, perhaps utilizing a genogram (Bowen, 1978; McGoldrick and Gerson, 1985), in a series of conjoint marital therapy sessions is useful for two reasons. First there is an opportunity to observe how the mates interact in examining material that is less threatening than current issues. Second, it gives the partners and the therapist an opportunity to see how they will work together and to develop a working alliance. Whether one uses a genogram or a series of questions to get the mates started talking or waits to see where they begin is less important than finding a way to assist their communication on issues other than the presenting problem once they begin talking.

THE SLOW PROCESS OF CHANGE

Healing occurs slowly. Therapists who have observed demonstrations of my work with narcissistically injured and vulnerable partners often comment upon the unhurried pace of the sessions, the repetitive patterns of interaction between the spouses, between each of them and me, and between the couple and me. The same expectations, demands and questions are raised over and over again. There is persistent pressure on both the partners and the therapist to react in a certain expected manner. The same buttons are pushed, the same hurts are inflicted, and the same reactions emerge—a hurried withdrawal or scathing rage. One spouse repeatedly turns to the other or to the therapist for confirmation that he or she is lovable, wonderful or special. When such confirmation is not immediately forthcoming in the prescribed manner, that spouse experiences deflation and disappointment.

Change is inhibited by the competing desire to maintain what is known, albeit painful. All living beings try to maintain the established order. Modifications do not occur at an even pace, nor does new cognitive awareness necessarily result in modification of destructive behavior. Only when new information is accepted and integrated into each partner's central organizing fantasy can there by any change in the emotionally shared experience.

It is tempting to try to right old wrongs by giving important others the power of early figures. When internalized conflicts from past family relationships are being relived in the present through the spouse and the children, treatment must include ways to understand the relationship between the intrapsychic and the interpersonal.

At first, integrating an awareness of what is occurring internally and interactionally is much more difficult for the couple than reacting immediately to the painful stimulus. The family system pushes against any decision to change and toward an effort to reestablish old patterns. The danger to the system feels real—an old fear that too great a change on the part of either mate can be overwhelmingly destructive. In response to the threat, the system tries to remain in homeostatic balance by reverting to past collusive interactions. Change can occur when, in a safe environment, partners begin to trust that the benefits of exploration outweigh the fear and the painful feelings.

As noted in earlier chapters, there is a tendency to organize experience within a personal framework that becomes an internalized model. A defense developed during the first years of life may have been the only response available to a young infant but can outlive its usefulness without itself being outgrown. When people who habitually employ primitive defenses marry, they relive, through the relationship with the spouse, the early fears and fantasies that first generated their defensive posture. We see this in the case of Roger and Rita.

Roger and Rita

After 12 years of marriage Roger decided to divorce his wife, Rita. "I don't want a mother," he proclaimed, as she verbally objected to being treated as his mother. "I let you do whatever you want. I offer you support and freedom to do what you wish. I don't know why you won't give our marriage a chance," she cried. Roger turned to the therapist, "I feel that she is manipulating me, that what she does for me is just meant to keep me trapped in this relationship. She is not doing it for me."

Responding to the therapist's question about whether he was reminded of any similar feelings in the past, Roger went on to talk of his parents' divorce. When he was three years old and his mother remarried, she and her new husband decided that they did not want Roger to live with them. He was "shipped off" to his father, who was also remarried and who soon sent him on to his grandmother. "I was a basket case by then. No one could handle me." He proceeded to describe years of living with a series of relatives and foster homes until the age of 18. At that point he left the midwest, where he grew up, and went to New York, where he became extremely successful in the theater.

At the age of 22 he married Rita, seven years his senior. For a few months he felt safe and knew that he had finally found someone who made him feel secure. But soon the old, upset feelings came upon him in waves of anger and mistrust. Whatever she did, it seemed upsetting. She was too close or too distant, too involved and smothering or too withdrawn, too demanding or too lenient with the children. Rita put her emotional energy into their two children and tried to make the best of the relationship. She was determined that her children not be part of a broken home as she had been. She did not want to end up divorced, like her mother and grandmother. But, the harder she tried to make the marriage work, the more he spoke of leaving.

Roger's wish to get away from Rita was based in part upon old feelings of anger and rage toward early caretaking failures and repeated abandonments. Rita could never provide him with enough to repair the old injuries—no one could. The pain that he lived with constantly could be mitigated by putting it somewhere outside himself. When he threatened to leave, his wife, rather than he, became the carrier of his abandonment fears. She was the frightened, upset child forced to share his pain by experiencing it herself.

We can see how the emotional failures in Roger's early interactions caused a lifelong inability to trust or feel secure in an intimate relationship. Almost from the beginning of his marriage Roger wanted to distance himself. Rita, meanwhile, was reexperiencing the old trauma of being abandoned when her father divorced her mother and disappeared. She was determined to save her children and herself from what she had come to expect would happen to her—that she, too, would be left. The harder she clutched to Roger, the more he pulled away.

It makes sense that the effects of early failures should be felt acutely in later attempts to establish meaningful long-term relationships. As Rita and Roger came to understand why their relationship had been feeling increasingly unsatisfying and dangerous, they stopped reacting in their repetitive push-pull manner. Each felt freer to stop at times and say that a specific interaction was extremely troublesome. They came to recognize that, as much as Roger pushed Rita away when she came too close, he desperately wished for the comfort of closeness.

Interestingly, a shift occurred in the relationship when Rita entered individual therapy and realized that she could, if necessary, survive without Roger. When he raised the spectre of divorce one day, Rita did not beg him to stay. She asked him how they would handle the business and financial arrangements. She talked of her intention of keeping the family home and asked if he had thought of where he might live. Had Roger truly wanted to leave he had his chance. Instead he suggested that they continue to work on their marriage in therapy and offered that he might benefit from some individual therapeutic sessions as well.

WHAT IS THERAPEUTIC IN THE THERAPEUTIC PROCESS

As we have seen, we cling to what is known and behave in ways that . confirm a particular world view. By selecting a mate whose inner world meshes more or less smoothly with our own personal framework, we are operating according to previously developed patterns and structures. Change in the ways that one feels, thinks or interacts requires a modification in the internal perception of the world and the self.

Pathology is a failure in the normal corrective process, an inability to use new information because of the defenses built earlier to protect the emerging self from maladaptive caretakers and from an environment perceived as hostile. The dangers against which the defenses have been erected usually remain unverbalized and out of the realm of our day-to-day awareness. Most of the time those things are not totally cut off or locked in the unconscious. Instead, they are given "selective inattention" (Sullivan, 1953), the habitual avoidance of potentially threatening experiences. Such adaptations are pathological to the extent that they preclude change and growth.

Early failures in interpersonal interaction may be mitigated by later relationships, including psychotherapeutic ones. Despite the anxieties that change arouses, the "working model" that develops early in life can be modified through experience. The term "working model" is used to imply that the internal images we carry around are not static. They are capable of change as new information is absorbed and new relationships offer the chance to repair preprogrammed expectations. If mother is unable to provide what the child needs, father may offer a compensating relationship. Siblings, peers, teachers and therapists can provide new reparative models. Change does not require conscious awareness, but a new way of interacting and responding that does not conform to old negative programming. Since models for behavior and emotional well-being are subject to positive feedback which amplifies new information, emotional development, even in adulthood, is a process of continuous change. The result of this process can become a corrective (Tolpin, 1983) or transformational (Bollas, 1987) experience.

Change may occur within either new or longstanding relationships when the other does not respond to some pressure to behave in an expected manner. The agent of change may be a therapist in an intense psychotherapeutic relationship or an intimate partner who chooses a reaction different from the ritualized reactions of the past, as Rita did with Roger. When his threats did not generate extreme anxiety in her, they were jointly able to reorganize some aspects of their relationship.

By helping a couple develop new responses to old stimuli, the therapist challenges them individually and collectively to arrive at a new construction of reality. It is fundamental that the individual clings to what is known; the grip must be loosened for him or her to grow and expand in the perception of self and others. While it is painful to have one's expectations violated, only through a positive response to such violations of expectations can one really change. The therapist assists by devising paths through which new information can enter, softening, but not erasing, the damage to each partner's expectations. Like any form of therapy, marital therapy proceeds in the faith that over time new ways of perceiving and being in the world can be developed. The difference between conjoint therapy and individual therapy is that in conjoint treatment the therapist is helping to change two individuals' sets of expectations and perhaps even a third—the set of expectations that constitutes the relationship itself.

In individual psychodynamic psychotherapy cure is attributed to the successful analysis of the transference relationship. Ideally, what the patient and therapist experience in the therapeutic relationship provides the analyst with a window into the patient's internal representations of the world of self and other. The therapist's nonjudgmental attitude and ability to contain and hold the patient's affect-laden reactions provide a benign atmosphere in which reactions and distortions that are inappropriate to the treatment situation may be examined as they are occurring.

Because the conjoint marital situation is not a totally accepting and benign atmosphere when partners are upset with and/or hostile to each other, it has been assumed that transference distortions cannot be re-examined. Furthermore, because the therapist takes a much more active role in the marital situation, it is thought to be more difficult to await the emergence of the transference or to reduce defensive reactions sufficiently to become aware of distortions in the interactions. However, I have not found it so. The active role of the therapist provides the boundaries needed to make the treatment a safe haven, to contain negative affects that invariably emerge, and to keep them from becoming destructive.

Early in marriage, partners typically attribute motivations to each other's behavior and communications that are not entirely accurate and probably do not represent the way the mate is experiencing the situation. As interchanges continue, the distortions build upon one another. Expectations of each other's negative reactions build into collusive interactions, and as time passes, the marriage is in trouble. Consequently, early in the relationship it is less difficult to correct distortions in interpersonal perceptions.

Jeanine and Marco

Jeanine became visibly upset every time Marco commented on her care of the house or her cooking. They had been married less than a year, and she believed that he was very sorry that the marriage had ever taken place. Her husband, a retired army officer, spent a lot of time "checking up on her housework." She came from what she called an "old-fashioned family," in which women "take care of their husband and children." Marco, almost 20 years older than she, said that he wanted to have children, but seemed so depressed that she assumed that he was thinking of leaving her.

Marco was a man of few words. After almost 30 years in the Army, he had retired and married for the first time. Marriage, he said, was all new to him. Retirement was also new. He did not know what to do with himself. He had lots of hobbies, but his life was not structured anymore. He had no idea that he was creating a problem for Jeanine, he said. He was just trying to keep her company. It concerned him that she didn't seem to want him around. He had begun to think that she was sorry that she had married a man 20 years older than herself. "Oh," replied Jeanine, "is that what was going on? You were worried about how I felt. I thought you were picking on me because you hated our marriage."

Jeanine and Marco were able to deal with their misperceptions before layers of bad feelings accumulated. However, when erroneous perceptions continue uncorrected over time, one sees mounting assumptions regarding intention and a tendency to build up barriers against being hurt by the other. When such perceptions recreate past emotional injuries, old and new interactions become confused and there is a buildup of defensive and retaliatory collusions.

Couples come into treatment with a full-blown transference that can be observed and utilized by the therapist trained to make use of such insights. It is the process of working through past patterns and their unconscious determinants, as well as actively seeking new responses, interactions and attitudes, added to the process of insight and understanding of transference and patterns of resistance, that is therapeutic in marital treatment. For therapy of any kind to be deemed successful, the individual or the couple must not only achieve a modification of perceptions and expectations, as well as increase in insight, but also develop a more satisfying relationship (Guttman, 1987).

An important aspect of work with couples involves getting them out of a purely preconscious, projective, introjective, collusive interaction into conscious understanding of their usual interchanges. As Skynner (1981) notes, the therapist's part in the process is to maintain the "parental holding role," keeping the situation constant and safe by providing a model of "play" (exploring, opening up, risking, venturing out into the unknown) and an attitude of certainty that gives hope of healing. The eventual goal is a change in which trust replaces distrust and understanding replaces misun derstanding, as both spouses realize that out of understanding comes giving.

In the process partners are aided in recognizing the emergence of repetitive collusive interactions and prepared to expect repetition of such reactions. When repetition occurs, they learn to observe carefully, perhaps even make notes about it afterward, and report to the therapist exactly what occurred. Making mental notes of the problem as it is occurring in order to report it in the therapy adds an observing ego to the interaction.

The therapist's role in marital therapy is to provide a holding space in which the marital partners feel safe enough to begin the process of re-owning the parts of themselves that they have denied, projected into the partner, and then defended against. As this re-owning takes place on a conscious level, partners show visible signs of relief. This relief comes about with the realization that each is now in control of the self and has a choice in how to express important issues consciously. There is a visible letting go of the spouse as an object of anger and fear.

LONG-TERM GOALS

In self psychology terms, a goal of psychotherapy for couples is increasing tolerance of selfobject (Kohut, 1977) failures so that they no longer cause fear of a loss of cohesion. The structures of the self may be developed to the point where there is a gradual maturation and evaluation of the selfobject needs and an internalization of selfobject functions. While that goal tends to be seen as requiring individual psychotherapy, I have worked with spouses who, through a willingness to allow each other to share heretofore cutoff aspects of themselves, have learned to relate to each other in an ongoing safe, nontraumatic environment with only occasional failures. These kinds of interactions provide opportunities for what Kohut (1971) calls "transmuting internalizations" to take place within the structure of the self. Transmuting internalizations are the changes that occur as the individual increasingly develops the capacity to accept the hurts that are caused by failures of important others to respond optimally. There is a gradually acquired ability to obtain from more varied sources the self-sustaining functions that previously had to be supplied via selfobject relationships. During the treatment process there is an awareness that the other is trying to hear and understand in ways that differ from the way he/she did it in the past. There is a willingness to acknowledge wounded feelings as they occur rather than cutting them off and retaliating. There is an increasing ability to recognize messages as meaning what the sender actually intended rather than resorting to automatic distortion. When there are provocations, attacks, or simply failures of needed responses, they can increasingly be tolerated, through facilitation by the therapist.

Howard and Lorraine

I include process notes from a session with Howard and Lorraine, a couple who have been married for six years and whose marriage reflects a history of past and current failures.

> HOWARD I know you want to have a family; so do I. But let's be logical. How can we start a family when we have so many financial problems? I am still trying to sell the business. I want to buy a ranch where it will be good to raise children.
>
> LORRAINE But I'm 35. I'm afraid it will soon be too late.
>
> HOWARD Lorraine, you haven't even said whether you are ready to move with me to the country.
>
> LORRAINE Well, it is far from all the friends I have made and from my work.
>
> HOWARD What does that mean—are you saying no, you don't want to move?
>
> LORRAINE I don't know.
>
> HOWARD How can you talk about having children when you may not even want to live with me?
>
> LORRAINE I wish you wouldn't get angry.
>
> HOWARD (more angrily) What do you expect! I try to plan with you rationally—and all you know is you want children. What about our lives together, what about my need to get away from the city?
>
> LORRAINE I guess a ranch might be all right. I never tried it. I won't know unless I try it.
>
> HOWARD So I'm supposed to move out to a ranch and have a baby and you'll let me know if you plan to stay—later. Well, no way am I going to be left with a child to support and a wife who can tell me she's leaving. First we will move and make sure it's working. Then we'll talk about children.
>
> LORRAINE I wish you didn't get so angry. It's not my fault that you have so many business problems.
>
> THERAPIST (I respond first to the conscious needs of each. Then I move to areas of vulnerability: e.g., Howard's need of an alter ego who thinks and wants what he does, and Lorraine's need of a soothing caretaking idealized other.) It sounds as though you know what you want, Howard, a home on a ranch with Lorraine

there with you. You get angry and upset when Lorraine says something that makes you feel that she wants things very different from what is important to you. (I then focus on Lorraine's fear of Howard's anger and her conscious attempt to do as he wishes to keep him from becoming angry at her.) And Lorraine, you seem to know what you want also—a family, a home. But when Howard gets upset, you become flustered. You don't know whether to stay with what you want or take care of Howard's upset feelings.

LORRAINE (responding first) I don't like Howard to get upset. When he does it makes me so upset and depressed. I just want to get away and hide. I feel like running away from home.

THERAPIST Does this remind you of feelings that you had in any past relationships?

LORRAINE It reminds me of how it was with my parents. I hated it when my father got so enraged and my mother went into a depression that made her act strangely for weeks. All of us kids tried hard to keep everything calm. (Lorraine gives some further information on her family history, a family in which mother's depressions and father's rages trapped the children into parentified caretaking roles.)

THERAPIST It must have been very hard to live there. Just as it's hard to live with Howard now. He tells you what he wants. You seem to be trying but sometimes you do what you want. Then he gets angry and feels left alone, not understood or cared for by you. I'm thinking of what you told me about your three brothers and sisters, who seem so tightly enmeshed in the family that they have never left their parent's home. You have proven you can leave and Howard has some concern that you will do just that. (I continue by focusing on Howard's part of the marital interaction.) Howard, I don't mean to speak for you, and I may be wrong. Please correct me if that is so. It seems to me that you keep telling Lorraine to leave when you get angry. But that is the exact opposite of what you want. You want her to want to be with you and show her love in ways that confirm that she understands your needs and feels as you do.

HOWARD That's right. Is that too much to wish for? She is my wife. What is good for me is good for her also.

THERAPIST The problem is that it leaves you always in a position where you are uncertain that Lorraine will be there. At any point she may want something different and fail to respond to your need. It makes you vulnerable to any signs that Lorraine's different wishes mean that she is withdrawing, abandoning you.

HOWARD Can anyone ever be sure? I was 40 when I married. Always I was careful because there is no guarantee that anyone will really be there for me. I guess that uncertainty is a part of living. That's why I make sure I can take care of myself and want Lorraine to be able to take care of herself.

THERAPIST I wonder about something when you say that. Stop me if I'm off base. It seems to me that neither of you has trouble taking care of yourselves. You both were well-functioning adults when you married. I think what you are talking about is what it means to be loved. Howard, you had some important losses when you were first learning about love. You said your mother was so involved in her charity and political causes that you had trouble getting her attention and your father often was at work until after your bedtime. And then he died when you were 12. I wonder if you ever had a feeling of someone being there for you emotionally.

HOWARD I knew they loved me.

THERAPIST How?

HOWARD I don't know. I know I was alone a lot. But when they were there I knew I could get attention. They took care of us, bought us what we wanted, at least until my father died. Then I was very depressed.

THERAPIST That's understandable. How about before? How did you get your parents' attention?

HOWARD I don't know. I know when I got angry about something they listened.

THERAPIST What kinds of things did you get angry about?

HOWARD I don't know. I don't remember—little things. (Momentary silence) I told Mom that I was sick—I had a sore throat. She didn't even take my temperature. She forgot, I think. I was seven or eight. I just stayed in bed that day. The housekeeper came at noon. She gave me some medicine. I was angry then.

THERAPIST Do you remember before that? Who was there for you?

HOWARD I remember when I was around three, I was alone with the babysitter. She had her boyfriend over and they locked themselves in a bedroom. I wished that God would send Mom home. I felt alone. Nothing happened. I stopped believing in God then.

THERAPIST It sounds as though your parents were busy people who weren't available to you—for whatever reason. When you needed them and didn't get what you needed you became very angry. Perhaps your surest connection with them was through anger. When it welled up they responded.

HOWARD I did used to get angry at them a lot when I was real young. But I outgrew it.

THERAPIST Do you remember when?

HOWARD By the time I became a teenager. I had my own friends. I didn't ask my mother for anything . . . except money. And my father was gone.

THERAPIST So, as you start talking about your history, it is not so unusual that you might become angry if you have a wish and Lorraine doesn't respond. You want someone to be there who will talk to you and respond to your needs. When you don't get it, perhaps anger is better than feeling the old desolation—the empty world without God or parents. When you are angry you make contact.

HOWARD (angrily) What do you mean—that I get angry at Lorraine to keep us talking?

THERAPIST Perhaps, and perhaps you push Lorraine away hoping that she will show you that she wants to be with you, as you need her to be.

LORRAINE But Howard calls me as often as I call him to make up after a fight. (Lorraine jumps in to protect Howard.)

THERAPIST (I recognize that I am pushing Howard perhaps too far and failing to be empathic. When confrontations or interpretations lead to resistance I recognize it as a failure of my function as a selfobject to the relationship. I turn to Lorraine to ask some questions about her history.) It may be, as it is with many couples, that fights for both of you are love signals that only sound like messages of anger. I wonder, Lorraine, if you had any early experiences similar to Howard's.

LORRAINE My family was pretty unusual. Everything looked good on the surface. Mom got spells when she was depressed but Dad was pretty levelheaded—except once in a while—he was like another person when he got angry. He'd scream and break things. But it didn't happen often. I never knew what set him off. I used to run into the bathroom and hide until he got over it. Sometimes Mom would come in and try to stop him. But that would only make it worse. But when he got over it, he became real nice. He held us kids in his arms. Sometimes he would cry and tell us he loved us.

THERAPIST You both had experiences in your life that help explain why you get into these fights that you think you don't want. Howard, you learned to get your needs for responsiveness met by getting angry. Any attention is better than busy, preoccupied parents. Even when you said you didn't care, you cared. We all need love. And when you tell Lorraine to go away, you don't need her, it is when you are aware of how much you do need her. You tell her to go and then want her back.

HOWARD She knows that I love her and don't want her to go. I guess I just overreact to some things.

THERAPIST Lorraine, you learned that you could get love after your father erupted spewing terrible stuff all around. Then he would hold you and reassure you of his love. Who knows what traumas in his life caused him to react that way. But you may have learned living in your family that it is possible to get love after an angry fight.

LORRAINE I don't know. Why would I do that—it hurts me so much when we fight. Even when we make up and everything is fine again, there is a piece of me inside that says, "Don't forget how much he hurt you."

THERAPIST You and Howard were not young when you married. You sifted through lots of prospective mates and found each other. Obviously there is a lot that's good as well as a lot that's difficult. We will have to look at both sides—what each of you needs and how you try to get the needs met.

In this case, Howard's need for a twinship relationship resulted in a particular collusive interchange with Lorraine. When she took an autonomous action that did not coincide with the intense needs or feelings that he was experiencing, he acted in ways that pulled her into his orbit. He did it by provoking in her a feeling of resourcelessness and anxiety about his rage. She responded with childlike helplessness and frustration and too much anger to think clearly. What she wished for was a warm, loving merger, a comfortable symbiosis. Each time Howard got angry, he destroyed a piece of her fantasy. Despite the problems that were produced by this pattern, Howard and Lorraine had essentially the same internal experience. The hateful arguments they had were designed to be a defense against a fragmented self caused by aloneness and emptiness.

Howard accepted the concept of female equality but based his insistence that they do things his way on two premises. The first was that she did not think logically and clearly, as he did. The second was that it was his business that gave them their lifestyle. He had all of the pressure to keep it going, and so it was her responsibility to put her energies into understanding and responding to his needs and into being available when he was free from his work. He experienced a particular type of merger expectation in the relationship, demanding that she be an extension of him—know his needs, think and feel as he did, and do nothing that would make him aware of their separateness. Whenever she did anything that confirmed the reality of her existence, that they were two separate people with their own individual needs and wishes, he became enraged.

When this illusion of oneness was broken, he would say, "What do I need you for? Get out of my life." When she went he found the aloneness unbearable and asked her to come back to try again. "Trying again" meant "Let's see if you can be a symbiotic extension of me." Lorraine had a complementary pathology that caused her to remain in and maintain the relationship. She had an unconscious wish to be taken care of totally by an ideal other—a combination husband, mother and father. She was prepared to submerge herself in an idealized other, just as she did in her family of origin.

Bollas (1987) notes that there are some patients whose goal it is to get under the skin of another, to coerce the other into experiencing resourcelessness and eventually a kind of hate. By doing so they form a negative selfobject, one constructed out of hate, but nevertheless one that yields a sense of intimacy, knowledge and safety. Howard and Lorraine fit this pattern. Howard's parents were largely unresponsive to his normal childhood desires, needs, aggressive feelings, or loving responses. Only through anger was he able to make a connection that he could believe in because he had some control. In that way hate can become a successful defense against separation and abandonment. Some persons hate the object not in order to destroy it but to preserve and maintain it. Hate does not emerge as a result of destruction of internal objects, but sometimes is a defense against emptiness (Bollas, 1983).

Lorraine similarly recognized the close connection between love and hate. Hateful attacks by her father preceded love and closeness. That made up for the desolation and emptiness she felt with her mother—a severely depressed woman who functioned within the family but rarely interacted with either the outside world or her children with any sense of intimacy or aliveness.

Marriages such as Howard and Lorraine's rarely change. They neither improve nor end. We continued working together for two months more. One day Howard asked me to validate his point of view in one of their disagreements. When I tried to interpret what he was doing, he demanded that I tell Lorraine how her behavior was the cause of their problems. I found myself frustrated and angry. I wondered if a confrontation would be the best approach. To Howard I pointed out that his demands made it difficult to proceed in our joint efforts to understand what was going on between them or to make lasting changes. At the same time I asked myself if his demands were designed to make our work impossible.

I had tried to make an interpretation without making a judgment that would create a narcissistic injury to this very vulnerable man. It did not work. He became angry at me and told Lorraine that they did not need this kind of help and that they were stopping treatment. She made no response. At the end of the hour they left.

When they stopped treatment I felt both sadness and relief. I went through a time of feeling that I had made a mistake and had failed them. Was there a way to avoid being caught in the pathological transference? Should I have tried more exercises or maintained firmer boundaries? Would another therapist have done it differently? Did I help them or simply add one more layer to the problem? As I mulled over these questions, I recognized that here, too, I was experiencing a piece of the uncertainty and anxiety that was so much a part of the marital system. I wondered if treatment would have been more successful if Howard or Lorraine or both had been in individual therapy. Because of their limited financial resources, they declined individual treatment. Yet, they needed it. I knew of no way of making such a suggestion at the time that they stopped treatment. Something would have to happen to interfere with their state of equilibrium—one in which passionate rage was a protection against the anxiety of aloneness and the fear of intimacy. I was surprised when, two years later, Howard called to ask for a referral to individual psychotherapy. Lorraine and the baby where doing fine, he reported, and he had decided that it was time to work on himself.

Once again, I recognized how much we do not know and that understanding alone does not cause change. Moreover, modification in a relationship does not necessarily result in the healing of the involved individuals' damaged structures. It is difficult to discern what experiences are being replayed endlessly, what defenses have developed and what they are designed to protect against. Insight into the etiology of a problem is, moreover, not sufficient to cause change. Partners may use such information against one another in a pattern of blame and shame. As we have seen, there are marriages in which both spouses have histories of severe psychological difficulties and yet appear to have a relatively conflict-free relationship, while other couples may show no evidence of individual pathology and yet be miserably unhappy.

In psychodynamic marital therapy, the marriage is the patient. In the consulting room, therefore, the therapist should convey a clear sense that the marriage is important, as are both people in it. The work between therapist and mates becomes an interactive process that provides clarity for the couple. One of the goals is to induce the spouses to regard the relationship as a center of empathic responses. Standing for the relationship, therefore, works two ways. In the beginning of therapy it takes the burden of defending or attacking the relationship off the partners, and later on it provides a reference point for work on empathic communication.

By acting in a manner that reinforces the safety and empathy required for successful conjoint therapy, as the interactive and intrapsychic process takes place, the therapist functions as a "holding environment" (Winnicott, 1971) for the marriage. This will be discussed further in the next chapter.

CHAPTER 9

Conjoint Therapy— A Safe Environment

When people are upset with or openly hostile to their partners, they frequently choose to be in individual therapy, where they may complain about the spouse. They are afraid that conjoint therapy cannot provide the empathic or containing environment needed for support. Many therapists assume that conjoint therapy is not an arena for psychodynamic change. Particularly with severely disturbed or narcissistically vulnerable patients, they assume that the only course of treatment is individual psychotherapy.

However, conjoint sessions provide both empathic understanding for the enhancement of a fragile self and a containing environment for the detoxification of dangerous projected internal representations. This is accomplished through therapeutic responses that focus not on the actions of each partner, but on the underlying affectivity that provokes negative actions and hostile reactions. Here I argue for the effectiveness of conjoint therapy in the treatment of marital problems. I will show how it works and how it uses the space established by the social nature of marriage. Because of this space, in some cases conjoint therapy can be more effective than individual therapy.

I will also show some specific ways in which the conjoint sessions can be utilized as an adjunct or alternative to individual sessions, particularly by becoming a holding environment in which dangerous affectivity that interferes in the relationship can be examined without producing overly intense anxiety or the emergence of self-protective defenses.

THE HOLDING ENVIRONMENT—
CONTAINER AND CONTAINED

In psychoanalysis the "holding capacity" of a therapist refers to the ability to remain constant, reliable, responsive, nonretaliatory, and relatively non-judgmental. The "holding environment" concept of Winnicott (1971), as well as Bion's "container" and "contained" (1970), suggests protection from overwhelming internal and external dangers.

Reliable holding, physical and emotional, must be a feature of the environment from the beginning of life for the development of a cohesive, enduring self. The integration of self and other and the development of the ability for relatedness both require "good enough" holding. The holding environment is a protection from physiological and psychological insult, and follows the day-to-day changes belonging to development. The matura-tional process is expedited by a facilitating environment (Winnicott, 1965). The early holding phase is equivalent to the stage of merger or total dependence, but the need for such holding recurs throughout life whenever there is a stress which threatens confusion or psychic disintegration.

The fantasy of many a new bride or groom is that marriage is such a holding place, a haven of safety in which occasional regression to depen-dence is tolerated, old injuries are repaired, and a barrier protects one from the dangers of the world outside. For a few the relationship becomes just such a holding place. For most, who unconsciously believe that falling in love means a lifetime of perfect happiness, the reality of a "good enough" marriage is a letdown. Romantic love promises more. It is the discrepancy between the idealized expectations of the loving, holding relationship, on the one hand, and the realities of maintaining a home, raising children, keeping jobs, and other aspects of living in modern society, on the other, that causes spouses to view each other as the cause of problems. Even as they each come to marital therapy filled with explanations of how the other must change, they fear being blamed. It does not occur to them that two people can be unhappy not because of the actions of one or the other, but because of the reactions of both to perceived injuries and expected threats. Each is reacting not only to the mate, but also to individual history.

In individual psychodynamic psychotherapy the therapist functions as a neutral sounding board and interpreter for the patient. By providing atten-tion, a nonjudgmental attitude, and an ability to contain the patient's affect-laden reactions, the psychotherapist offers a benign atmosphere in which reactions, distortions, and feelings can be examined as they occur. In that way, whatever is experienced within the therapeutic relationship becomes a window into the internal world of the patient.

The goal of the therapist is to make sessions a holding space, an island of safety. That requires the establishment of an environmental container where boundaries are carefully delineated. To make therapy such a holding space, where it is safe to bring old frightening feelings and reactions to the light of day, the therapist must hear and understand the underlying messages of both partners.

When a person is seen only in individual treatment, the emotional injuries and acting-out on the part of a partner may be seen as indicative of a pathological and perhaps irreparable marital relationship. Certainly each mate may have cause to feel victimized by the other. Therapy is often seen as a time to treat individual problems that caused failure of a marriage. If it is thought that there were unconscious reasons for selection of a mate based upon similarities of pathology (Dicks, 1967; Gurman, 1979), then treatment may become focused on disentanglement from a destructive relationship and avoidance of such a pathological relationship in the future. But many apparent pathological interactions in relationships are dyadic in nature, with action and reaction building upon each other with increasing damage to the relationship. Conjoint sessions that provide a container for underlying vulnerabilities and pathological defenses may allow for discussion of shameful or humiliating reactions associated with vulnerabilities and defenses, thereby enabling the couple to disentangle from collusive interactions while remaining in the relationship.

INDIVIDUAL SESSIONS
IN MARITAL THERAPY

Many therapists who work with couples give examples of successful outcomes combining ongoing individual treatment of one or both partners with conjoint sessions. In attempting to resolve issues that interfere with a relationship, I may occasionally have individual sessions as needed. I have, however, found such sessions less necessary as I have learned new ways to work with the couple conjointly. Certainly, if individual sessions can help the partners to clarify thoughts and understand better what they wish to express to each other, they can be of value, but there is a danger in allowing them. Partners may vie to be the therapist's favorite or incorrectly report what occurred in the individual sessions. Or one partner may choose to share a secret about an affair that potentially puts the therapist in the position of colluding to hide important information. Therapists differ in the way they handle secrets. Some insist that all secrets are open for discussion in the conjoint sessions at the discretion of the therapist. Others say up front that nothing will be shared by the therapist regarding individual sessions. I prefer the latter; nothing said in the individual sessions is raised as an issue by me in conjoint sessions.

If in an individual session one partner wants to tell me such a secret, the more important question at the moment is: What does he or she wish to achieve? Is it a need to unburden on someone who will listen—or is it a desire to have a "therapeutic affair," a collusion between us that leaves the partner out of *our* secret alliance? The reason may be more important than the secret for the purpose of diagnosing and treating the marital pathology.

When I accept a case for marital treatment, I advise the couple that I see the marriage as the focus of the treatment. One goal of our work together is to see that individual problems do not do further damage to the relationship. Another is to assure that the marriage does not intensify individual problems. Although the treatment may very well help them resolve long-standing psychological vulnerability, the focus at the beginning of treatment is on changing destructive marital interactions.

BOUNDARY ISSUES IN THERAPY

Many couples have problems with boundaries—inside and outside the self, and between self and other. When people marry and hear the words "two people become one," the narcissistic message is "I am the one." Some narcissistic individuals assume that the mate will now function as an extension, an additional arm, to do and think as an identical twin might. Others, whose narcissistic injuries occurred at the point of declaration of autonomy, and may still be fighting to have a self and will see danger in any boundary merger. They are considered "commitment shy"; even after marriage they make clear their need to maintain a separate space and to have time to be away from the relationship.

It is necessary to understand boundary issues in order to avoid the presumption of pathology where there are actually differences of boundary needs. Some couples are happy twosomes who merge boundaries, rarely disagree on issues, finish each other's sentences, and feel quite safe immersed in one another. Others are convinced that opening the boundaries of the self will lead another to attempt to control them. Where pathology and defenses underlie individual behavior, the lack of differentiated boundaries results in what Bowen (1972) described as an "undifferentiated family ego mass," in which both spouses and children are pulled into pathological family interactions.

For example, Bud insisted on going out with his single friends to sports events and on playing poker one night a week. Laurel said that she would love to learn more about sports and that she likes to play poker. She felt unloved and rejected when he appeared cold to her suggestion that she join him and his buddies in his activities. Bud felt his wife trespassing on his private space and withdrew. Not until they came to understand their different expectations about boundaries and needs could they work out a closeness-distance pattern that was acceptable to both.

The therapist must know the different ways that individuals and couples deal with boundary issues. Figure 9.1 identifies some boundary differences in narcissistic interactions.

There is a maturation in all human beings along developmental lines in

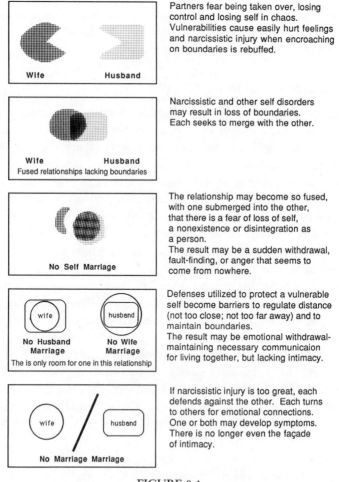

FIGURE 9.1
Boundary Differences in Narcissistic Interactions

such important areas as affective experiences, consolidation of the self, emotional connection of the self with others, and acquisition of words, symbols and thought patterns. Where the early environment did not provide a container to safely allow affects, emotion, thoughts and feelings to emerge, pathological conditions develop. The result may be a lifetime of searching for a containing environment to provide both the initially needed responses and an opportunity to reexperience reflectively or behaviorally the reactions to early failures. It is when there is a deeply felt lack of such that mates may reach across boundaries in an attempt to acquire what is needed.

NONVERBAL INFORMATION

The joint work involves understanding the "non-understandable" and making reason of the apparently unreasonable (Giovacchini, 1987). For example, why does one partner flare up in rage at a certain message? Why does one refuse to discuss a particular subject? It is important for the therapist to recognize that the patient's behavior makes sense in some context, that it is quite reasonable behavior, considering the history of the individuals, development of the relationship, and current circumstances that have led to the immediate problem. To discover the meaning of seemingly unreasonable reactions is not the same thing as endorsing them. It is an attempt to bring to awareness and verbalize deep layers of affective experience.

Much information that is significant to the marital relationship is never overtly stated by partners to each other. Nevertheless, conscious and unconscious material that is not verbalized is acted upon by one or both partners. When nonverbalized messages are understood and presented in a nonjudgmental manner in the safe relational space of a therapeutic session, it becomes possible to examine them for underlying meanings. The need to defend a vulnerable self and the need for affirmation to enhance the self are among the most important underlying causes of apparently unreasonable behavior. It is often a great relief to both partners when emotions and affects related to these needs are examined in a neutral environment.

Such information can be presented gently as a hypothesis to be examined and affirmed or discarded as incorrect or premature. Some important messages, based upon lifelong patterns of reacting to significant others, are sent and received between partners through mutually reinforced projective or introjective patterns. The content of these messages, so basic to the interactions in any intimate partnership, can be inferred by listening to the communication process of the couple after the initial presentation of the problem. The chief themes are stated early. The dynamic of the dyadic interaction then emerges and becomes available for the working-through process.

Reaching this state requires a haven of safety for the therapeutic exploration of the damaged structures of the self, as well as a change in the interactions that are in place to protect the vulnerable self from further injury. Changing defensive collusions requires the courage to face up to the shadows and ghosts that reside in the current relationship. If the mates can accept each other as they are and share the unresolved residue of the past in each other's presence, then they may be able to come close enough to share a future of intimacy.

REDIRECTION OF PROJECTIONS

Almost by their nature too-painful feelings must be split off, denied, and dumped into any handy container. Because of their proximity, family members all too often become those containers. I do not believe that narcissistic individuals are attempting to damage the receivers of their toxic projections. The projection starts as a wish for a fairy godmother—someone to receive unbearable affect, take custody of the feelings for a while, clean them and return them nicely detoxified. While their feelings are out there, while they are raw and dangerously vulnerable, individuals want someone to say soothing, reassuring words—something, of course, that is not likely to occur in the normal course of human relationships. So other things happen to the projections. The therapist must watch for the transformation of the projection from a cry for help to an attack. The spouse receiving the projection quite likely has become accustomed to being bombarded with unacceptable feelings, without knowing how it happens. When the communication seems designed to provoke a reaction, the form of intervention involves listening to a piece of the interactive process, then asking for clarification. Afterwards, it is possible to make interpretations about the vulnerable feelings that caused a need for defensive projections.

When projections occur the therapist may ask the spouses to stop for a moment and examine exactly what provoked the interaction. If the interaction is based upon blame or attack, the same process is used as a redirectional experience. For example, such a redirection begins with an empathic response to each person, a careful listening to overt complaints, underlying affectivity, and defensive postures, and then their translation into needs, fears, and hurts. The therapist may direct a generalized statement to the husband, such as, "When a person is hurt, he is likely to defend himself," and to the wife, "When a person feels misunderstood or attacked, the defense may take the form of a retaliatory attack." The spouses are asked how they defend against such hurts from each other. In the process it is possible for defenses to be understood and accepted, for toxic projections to be contained, held with care, and returned detoxified. The work of the therapist is to accept and tolerate what the fragile self finds intolerable and the mate considers unacceptable or "crazy." After a period of time the toxic projections may be redirected back where they originated, but in a manner that does not raise more anxiety than the partners or the marriage can stand.

Handling projections requires going back and forth between partners, allowing anxious feelings to emerge without being pushed away or projected for as long as the partners can tolerate. The therapist speaks with each mate and attempts to determine what predisposed one or both to such strong defensive needs—what hurt so much? Such exploration may include examining early formative experiences, allowing for the emergence of the anxiety, sadness, or anger that underlies the development of the defensive position.

The therapist acts as a container, taking in whatever is "dumped," whether it is accepted or deflected by the partner. By absorbing the blaming behavior—the projected affect—the therapist prevents feelings from being cut off and denied. They are allowed to remain in the therapeutic environment and are drawn upon for help in understanding the couple's collusive system.

What is learned by the couple in treatment is that heretofore dangerous interactions can now come up without being destructive to the relationship. The anxiety and pain may still be there, but, with the therapist to assist in holding the frightening feelings, there is an increasing ability to tolerate them.

George and Eva

George and Eva had spent the four years of their marriage continually on the verge of separation and had twice before tried to work out their difficulties in therapy. Each time therapy was terminated when the therapist focused upon George's pathological reactions and seemed to be encouraging Eva to end a relationship that appeared to be so damaging to her.

Each had strengths, talents, and high intelligence, and yet from the beginning of the treatment there were signs of a frightening intensity of affect lying just below the surface of both partners and of their relationship as well. Each partner presented a history of family disruption and chaos. At an unconscious level both were seeking a place to hold a deep disturbance. The countertransference reactions, which will be discussed later, and their responses when I took their history gave many clues to their individual and joint difficulties.

George had a traumatic childhood, growing up in a home that revolved around religious fanaticism and the care of a seriously ill younger child. He was a misfit in school and misunderstood at home. Sometimes, he said, he felt crazy, but he drew upon an inner strength to survive emotionally. He had the talents and abilities to achieve goals that he set for himself, yet he always felt a sickness lurking below. His life and his relationships were a constant battle. His relationships were never true connections, he said.

Eve described a childhood experience of moving from a very poor home with her mother to an upper-middle-class neighborhood with her mother and new stepfather. The cultural shock of entering a new socioeconomic group with a different ethnic background from hers made her feel stupid and inadequate. The educational system was more advanced than the one she came from; moreover, the other children made fun of her because she spoke with the accent of her old community. She also had been poorly prepared for the intense competition to excel among students in her new school and had to work extremely hard just to keep up. She never realized how bright she was during all of her growing-up years. Her negative feelings about herself were exacerbated by her stepfather's dislike of her and by her being sexually molested by a relative over a period of time.

Eva seldom talked as a child. She was shy, did not cause trouble in school, and was hardly noticed by the teachers. She tried to hide her accent by hiding her words. She retaught herself to speak without an accent but had to be careful to never speak too spontaneously or she might forget herself and fall back into her old way of talking. No matter how much she learned or achieved, she was left with a feeling that her true self was hidden away and what the world saw was a façade, a necessary cover-up. She lived in terror that something would cause her carefully constructed world to fall apart.

As an adult she took a job that made demands well below her actual abilities; she found herself teaching and helping others at work but not getting the help, support, and encouragement she was seeking. When she told her husband of her frustrations at work, he said she was too good for the job and advised her to quit. She resisted that solution and held on to her secure employment with a tenacity that he did not understand. When he proceeded to give her other advice she got angry at him. They lived through a series of escalating battles in which he screamed and she withdrew.

George experienced a growing feeling of inadequacy to help her. He kept trying to find an answer to make her feel better so she would stop being so upset. He needed her to be the strong competent person he believed her to be. Unconsciously her role was to function as a container of his affect—to make him feel he would not be abandoned when he was not fully in control of his emotions. Each was seeking in the other a solid, stable "mother representation" who would repair an early defective care-taking experience.

When George could not get Eva to feel better, he became enraged. Eva responded by becoming frightened of a reaction which seemed to be full of hate, and she withdrew from him. Not only did she not get the support and comfort she sought, but she got instead an angry, frightened and frighten-ing man. She did not understand his transition from a highly competent, rational husband to a screaming, irrational creature.

Eva felt that she had no control in the relationship and considered leaving George. She went into therapy, where she discussed her problems and frustrations. Her therapist thought that she could never grow and develop as an independent, autonomous person as long as she was married to George. She stayed in the marriage and left the therapy. Certainly, the marriage could have been seen as a mutually collusive relationship in which the termination of individual treatment reflected a resistance to growth. However, when the couple later requested conjoint therapy, they identified from the beginning individual problems that were interfering with the relationship and did not blame or attack each other as such spouses often do. Treatment was undertaken on this basis.

In therapy George investigated his own frightened reactions to his loss of control. He spoke of feeling crazy. He mentioned having psychotic reac-tions in his adolescent and young adult years—and of growing up in a cult-like family in which much of what was going on made no sense. He lived in a world at war, in which bombs, death, good and evil were part of daily life, and in which he had real fears of his own destruction. He studied and learned to become a leader among his siblings, and later, in his community, but he always felt that beneath the façade of strength was a core of dangerous craziness.

As he related his history, he connected his early upbringing to the dysfunctional way that he lived his adult life. He married young and had a child. He could not tolerate it when the baby cried, to the point of fearing that he might hurt or kill the child. Long after his divorce and remarriage to Eva he continued to feel a great discomfort about his reactions. For this reason he would not consider having another child, fearing the "devils" inside him. As he described these frightening reactions, he seemed to carefully parcel out his emotions in order to protect his wife and the therapist from the "unbearable." As he spoke of his archaic emotions, he recognized that his reaction to Eva when she was upset resembled both the feelings he had had toward his baby and his own childhood rages. In each case the intensity of affect could be traced to a sense of having lost control over his situation, and in each case he reacted by losing control of himself.

Over a period of months he repeatedly mentioned the battles between his irrational rage and his thinking self. His wish to share openly the secret shame of murderous impulses was clear. He wanted them to be heard by his wife and by the therapist. They were not unconscious feelings; they were known but rarely allowed into the realm of conscious thought. Primitive chaotic affects that were unacceptable and hidden away were beginning to be recognized and identified in words. He was clearly relieved at being able to talk about his troubling thoughts and feelings, and Eva was relieved that she could understand his behavior. Once the process of communicating and being understood began, a deep well of emotions arose.

George and Eva began to react toward each other in a new way when problems arose. This couple had, fortunately, much more to them than their areas of pathology. There was intelligence, a sense of humor, and a reservoir of caring and goodwill for one another. It was hard not to admire their shared determination to resolve their severe individual and mutual pathology.

As the therapy progressed, they became increasingly aware of a lightening in their individual problems. By working conjointly, each became responsive to the other. Each learned what hurt the other, what would help, and how to be available. They learned that they could get their needs met by one another outside of the therapy hour and were increasingly willing to be a container to each other. In treatment they both came to realize that what Eva wanted from George was not advice or suggestions, but to be listened to, acknowledged for her anxiety and needs, and reassured of his love.

The therapeutic role throughout this process was to make the sessions a place where feelings and fears could be identified and dangerous impulses explored. We focused on examining how feelings arose in interactions in the past, what brought them up in the present, how they affected a current relationship, and how the feelings were contained, split off, or otherwise defended against.

CONTAINING ANXIETY

From the start the therapist lets the couple know that the goal is to understand as nearly as possible the needs of each partner, the things that bring on emotional pain, and the way that each defends vulnerable areas.

When needs, hurts, or defenses come up in the sessions, they are viewed not as problems, but as opportunities for exploration. Issues of living are dealt with unless or until an area of narcissistic need, injury, or defense arises. At that point, we temporarily put aside whatever is being discussed to make the therapeutic setting a container for the anxiety that inevitably emerges and prepare to examine how a specific issue becomes part of the partners' collaborative dance.

The dance begins when the partners meet and select each other. The initial choice of a mate has much to do with the match of unconscious "programs" carried over from the early decisions made in the interactions with parents, as we saw in Part One. Through projective defenses it is possible to split off internalized unacceptable impulses and feelings and hand them over to a mate who more or less willingly accepts them. The wish is to contain anxiety and alleviate intense emotions.

It is a challenge, as every therapist knows, to help those who utilize primitive defenses. In conjoint therapy, the process may include allowing the partner or therapist to take on projections in collusive patterns, intervening at appropriate points in the collusions that invariably arise, asking how the difficulty is usually played out in the real environment outside of treatment, and directly examining with the couple how the usual reaction of each provokes vulnerable areas within the other.

Within the atmosphere of a containing therapeutic environment, the therapist may stop the process when things begin to warm up, tell the partners that they are getting to the heart of something that hurts them both a great deal, and suggest that they try to stay with what they feel as they speak and listen to each other. When there is an attempt to avoid, change the subject, or attack the other, the therapist redirects: "I know what just happened must be very painful. What do you usually do when it feels too awful to tolerate?" Responding to the pain with empathy, rather than responding to the issue precipitating the overwhelming affect, often reduces anxiety and allows the person to examine the cause of the burning feelings. The mate is then asked, "What feelings do you have that correspond with what you just heard? How do you defend against your too painful feelings?" The discussion then focuses on the feelings themselves rather than on the issues the mates usually fight about.

This can lead into a discussion of how each perceives the other's feelings and behaviors, how much they were aware of before this discussion, and what they generally do when such feelings come up in their lives together. The therapist is then in a position to show how each partner's usual defenses, which feel to the other as attacks or withdrawals, are meant to protect a vulnerable self.

Robert and Ada

Robert's usual blustering rage at what he perceived as the failure of his wife, Ada, to manage the children and their home was intercepted during one fiery outburst. "I know it is upsetting to hear that her job will take her out of town on the day of your son's Little League championship game," I commented, "but you seem more than upset. You look as though you could kill. It's more than the game, more than the job. There's something about her not paying attention, not seeming to care. Can you help me to understand what it touches inside of you, what it reminds you of?"

Robert responded with a poignant account of his experience growing up during the Korean War years. With his father in the service and his mother preoccupied with work, he had learned not to expect anyone to come to special events in school or to share the excitement of Little League games. It hurt to see the same thing happening to his children. Even as I encouraged Ada and Robert to discuss the issues, and the intensity calmed down enough to consider some alternatives, it felt as though the rage was disproportionate to the precipitating source. I weighed the possibilities that the real problem was Robert's overidentification with his son as a Little League star, his jealousy of his wife's career success, or his intolerance of being alone when Ada went on a business trip. Recognizing that issues that arise and remain unresolved without being experienced as a threat or attack are likely to resurface at a later time, I said nothing, and waited to learn more.

Soon afterward, the same problem emerged in the context of an argument over a male co-worker. It felt to Robert as though the man was paying too much attention to Ada. At an office party he had invited Ada to dance. Robert left the party in a rage. Ada cried as we talked about it, but Robert was still angry. I told him, "I can see how angry you are right now, but I need you to hold onto the feeling for a moment, so that I can also understand what Ada is feeling." I kept it short at this point because I knew that Robert could only hold his anger for a moment. Ada, still crying, explained how Robert shamed her in front of her co-workers. She was only trying to be pleasant to the new management trainee in the office. He had been there for a week and didn't know many people. I responded, "The embarrassment and anger that you felt have not gone away. You seem still very upset right now."

Ada's response was, "I'm terrified that he is going to hit someone again." I turned to Robert and said, "It sounds as though you have tried hard to control your anger, but have not always been successful. Whom did you hit?" Robert and Ada then proceeded to tell me of an incident shortly after their marriage when an old boyfriend of Ada's came over to their table in a restaurant and began talking. At one point he had put his arm around her shoulders and gave her a hug, Robert, unable to contain himself, got up and punched the man. Robert said, "It never happened again, and it will never again." Ada responded, "I don't know if I can believe you." Robert seemed transformed into a pose of humiliating capitulation. Ada was right not to trust his temper. For the moment she had control of the situation. I turned to Ada and said, "I do not know if Robert will ever hit someone again in a jealous rage, but the rage is still there and we better understand what that is all about."

I did not confront Robert directly with an expectation that he would explain his feelings. Rather, still facing Ada, I asked, "Does either of you know anything about your histories that would shed some light on his feeling that you are not to be trusted, that you might want to be with another man?" With some hesitation, Robert related that his mother had had a lover while his father was in Korea. The man had lived with the two of them in their small apartment. Robert, who was six at the time, knew that there was something wrong with the man's sleeping in his mother's bedroom. Then, suddenly, after weeks or months, Robert could not recall, "Uncle Charlie" was gone. By Christmas his father was home. His mother had warned him never to mention Uncle Charlie's visit. When he asked why not, she said that, if Robert told, his father would leave and would never come back: "You don't want Daddy to leave forever, do you?"

Robert choked up and was unable to go on. I said, "There are many tears that go with that story. You have never had a chance to shed them. What you've done is put your memories in a box and locked them up. When something comes up in your life that pushes the combination to the lock, all the confused, hurt, angry and frightened feelings that you couldn't feel then erupt at one time. And it all gets directed at Ada. I can see how the two of you have had so much trouble."

The fear of being "found out" is mixed with the wish to be understood at the deepest levels of one's being. When words are put to those things that are known deep within the self but had been kept out of the realm of consciousness, a feeling of relief is quickly recognized, both through body posture and through the newfound ability to continue to talk. When it becomes clear to both partners that their underlying messages will be heard, at least by the therapist if not initially by their partner, it is possible for them to learn different ways of responding. The initial anxiety that each experienced upon entering therapy quickly fades and turns to a safe, containing, contextual transference.

REACTION TO THE THERAPIST

By providing a safe environment for old, frightening feelings and reactions, the therapist changes the pattern of interaction between partners. Despite his or her efforts to maintain a nonjudgmental neutrality in communication with couples, the therapist will often be perceived as taking sides or as being hurtful in other ways. When that occurs, the therapist can hear what is not said through observing the body language of the partners, and by paying attention to his or her countertransferential reactions. If the therapist feels tired, distant or anxious, for example, something is going on between or among the partners and the therapist.

If either partner reacts as if the therapist is aligning with the other, whether or not it is based on a correct perception, the focus must shift away from the interaction between the spouses to that between the therapist and one or both of the spouses. For example, it is possible to say to one partner, "I feel as though I am missing something that's important to you. I wonder if we can stop for a moment so you can tell me if I am hearing you wrongly or hurting you by what I am saying," or, "You seem to be very distant today—I wonder if something that is happening here is making you upset or angry."

If the person says, "I'm just tired today" or "I'm worried about work," the therapist may still consider the possibility that what is happening relates to the therapy. People who spend the time and money to see a marital therapist want help with their relationships. When they react in the sessions in a manner that says they are upset, they very well may be upset with the session or with what happened in past sessions.

Whatever the response is at that point, the therapist's initiation of a confrontation is likely to make the person withdraw. Rather, the therapist should respond by saying something like, "I just wanted to check, as I know that some issues cause great pain and hurt to people and I don't want to push forward in an area that causes too much discomfort. Our work is to make clearer what has gone wrong—not to add blame to the problems you already have." By giving careful regard to each partner's fear of being abandoned or blamed by the therapist, the therapist helps the spouses to focus inward and move away from the nonproductive pattern of projective blaming and projective identification.

As the underlying messages are conveyed between partners through the therapist, several important messages are being sent. Although there is wish to be infallibly correct, our interpretations and interventions sometimes miss the mark. When someone feels misread, it is important to offer an opportunity to correct and challenge what is said. Both the content and the form of a challenge can, in fact, provide important clues about the message and the messenger. A comment delivered in a tone that chokes off rage can be very informative, for example. When either partner does not seem to feel accurately understood, the therapist has a direct opportunity to clarify the situation. Once again, the attempt to communicate, in addition to addressing the immediate issue, models something very important, because the partners experience attempts by another person at empathic under-standing of their messages. That the attempt is not successful is sometimes not as important as the fact that the attempt was made at all.

THERAPEUTIC NEUTRALITY AND THE ISLAND OF SAFETY

Some family therapists use interventions that contradict projected expecta-tions in order to break up an established pattern. I am not a believer in "shocking the family into a high level of heightened awareness and so out of their dreams and self-fulfilling negative prophesies" (Skynner, 1981, p. 72). Instead, a treatment approach should center on making therapy a safe haven where responses that would normally cause embarrassment or hu-miliation can be brought into conscious awareness and discussed openly. That includes helping partners recognize and talk about their own fearful, shameful, or hostile reactions. In the safety of the treatment environment there is an effort to mitigate the unsettling effect such talk can have. Discussion diminishes the repetitive, collusive interactions meant to keep both partners in the dark about vulnerable areas, thus making their de-fenses less necessary.

To create a feeling of safety, the therapist should be prepared to go along with the couple as a guide, not as an all-knowing expert. We all make mistakes and acquire knowledge. The therapist must be as interested in his or her own reactions in the session as in the reactions of the individual or couple. These reactions may involve the unpleasant and frightening—loss, separation, death, sexuality, and competitiveness. Sometimes it is possible to share feelings with clients before those feelings are fully understood and integrated. Some significant therapeutic impasses have been broken down when I have risked sharing with a couple somewhat unthought-out and yet intuitively known feelings (Bollas, 1987). This will be discussed further in Chapter 11.

As therapy progresses, the partners begin to communicate with each other about things that had been considered too dangerous or embarrassing to say. Hurt and dependency may be admitted as the spouses improve their ability to function as selfobjects for each other. Together they begin to develop a quid pro quo: "I will not attack you in your vulnerable areas if I have some assurance that you will not try to hurt me when I show my vulnerabilities." Both recognize that this is not an easy goal to achieve, and failures do occur as they try to communicate in greater depth with each other. As they learn to reduce the areas in which they hurt each other, and each recognizes the intent of the other as a wish to understand and be responsive, failures do not result in immediate defensive measures. Slowly, the structures of the self develop more tolerance for the missed response. The process is similar to what Kohut (1977) called "transmuting internalization."

The goal is to encourage self-observation and self-understanding when hurt, anger, or humiliation arises in interactions. Rather than blaming the other, self-awareness is stimulated in each partner. The redirection of the traditional pattern of the couple frees the relationship and allows the partners to proceed with the work of addressing unfinished business. "The therapist's final effort is to help each spouse develop a greater awareness of his or her individual issues which feed the marital conflict" (Beck, 1987, p. 157). The ultimate result might be initiation of individual therapy, group therapy, or a continuation in conjoint therapy with the couple functioning as a small psychotherapy group.

In some instances the combined effort of husband, wife and therapist may provide a holding environment for intolerable feelings. The partners may utilize the marital system as the contextual environment in which there can be a reactivation and a healing of those aspects of the core self that had been damaged (Scharff and Scharff, 1987). Major change in defensive maneuvers can be accomplished in the working relationship of a long-term treatment that encourages growth and change in each of the partners.

Ultimately, the goal of marital therapy is not only to promote a greater degree of empathy in the relationship, but also slowly to rebuild the structures of the self. Each partner comes to trust the marital relationship and the therapy as a safe environment where intense feelings, such as frustration and rage, may be experienced without fear of devastation and destruction, and where emptiness and numbness can be identified without shame. The partners learn new ways to respond to each other constructively, and they then use this knowledge to enhance their life between sessions and upon termination.

CHAPTER 10

Multilevel Communication

Spouses having marital problems are not good at translating each other's messages accurately. It is as though they speak different languages. They are too vulnerable and there is too much "noise" in their interactions. It is difficult for them to make themselves understood because the language of feelings and needs is rarely spoken directly, appearing instead in encoded form. One must have both an understanding of the other's language and a willingness to hear it in order to decode it properly. It is at this level that a dynamically oriented psychotherapist can be of great assistance to individuals who are trying to improve their relationships.

At all times the therapist monitors the discussion to be sure both partners are involved. "Involved" does not necessarily mean "talking." It means that the one communicating really knows that the other partner is attending. "When the therapist succeeds in facilitating an open congruent expression of vulnerability from a blaming hostile spouse, followed by an accepting response from the other, withdrawn spouse, a new kind of interaction cycle becomes possible" (Johnson, 1987, p. 72).

If a relationship has had a pattern of repeated injuries, there is little goodwill between the partners and limited trust at the onset of treatment. They begin with a combination of hope and anxiety, often a belief that they must be prepared to defend themselves against being blamed for the marital problems. As we have seen in the last chapter, the therapist functions as the container of dangerous communications between partners. There is little advantage in the therapist's simply advising partners to talk directly to each other when the history indicates that their communication is utilized as a means of attack and defense. A new language must be learned.

This chapter will discuss the various levels of messages, unspoken and spoken, intended and unintended, conscious and unconscious, direct and manipulative. It is not unusual for people to send messages at many conscious and unconscious levels at the same time. "Of all of the marvels in human communication, perhaps the most awesome is the ability of the human mind to express itself simultaneously on two distinct and yet interconnected levels of meaning" (Langs, 1983, p. 3). Possibly, the recognition skills that reside at such deep nonverbal levels are related to methods of communication developed by the human species before the advent of language. The unconscious sharing of affect provides alternative routes for the communication of internal states.

THE MANY LANGUAGES OF MARITAL INTERACTION

In our culture, heavily laden with linear thinking and rational modes of viewing the world, there tends to be an assumption that truth is based upon that which is consciously known, identifiable, and measurable. The scientific method follows the principles of logic, observation, testing and replication to confirm reality and truth. But truths are relative to the questions asked, the instruments of measurement, and the contextual meaning of the message. What we think is limited by the tools we have for conscious thought—words and symbols. These limits may be expanded by reaching into other realms of communication, such as art, music, poetry, and folklore. What is spoken carries multiple levels of conscious and unconscious communication. What a therapist listens for are the messages that come from defenses and from underlying needs.

While it is impossible to communicate at all operative levels at once, it is similarly impossible not to communicate—even silence is a communication (Watzlawick, Beavin, and Jackson, 1967). A simple question, such as, "Do you need my help?" may include such nonstated messages as, "I want you to appreciate me, . . . notice me, . . . need me, . . . love me, . . . forgive me."

As noted earlier, everyone protects vulnerable areas by using various defenses. Messages about needs, fears, and emotions are sent in ways that cannot be consciously understood by most of those around us. Partners in intimate relationships, however, have many ways of recognizing and understanding such unconscious communication—ways that to an outsider might seem almost like psychic phenomena.

In fact, if communication were limited to what is accessible to conscious awareness and can be verbally communicated, relationships would be dull, empty, and lifeless. To be filled with energy, intimate interactions must go below the single, surface meanings into the underlying, multileveled, encoded communication of the whole self. Some couples can communicate quite well about maintaining a household, functioning of social engagements, and arranging schedules for their children, while their relationship is barren and unrewarding to each.

Communication is, thus, a combination of conscious and unconscious encoding. Messages sent and received may be logical or illogical, clear or disjointed, congruent or incongruent. Direct messages can appear to be sensible and logical, while hidden meanings, sometimes contradictory, are presented in understandable and readable form to the other person. "We find those messages that have imaginative surface implications and several levels of easily sensed (if difficult to define) underlying encoded meanings especially exciting and provocative. Therein lies the beauty of . . . an exquisite and unforgettable moment of love" (Langs, 1983, p. 15).

Messages do not exist in limbo. Within the context of a relationship the receiver hears the subtle undertones that validate or confirm the meanings at the surface level and illuminate the underlying wishes, needs, fears and defenses. The context includes not only the here and now of the sender and the receiver of the communication, but also the entire history of each person and the particulars of the relationship and the setting. Each partner has an internal world of object representations of self and other. Each has split-off aspects that are communicated not in words, but in nuances that communicate with the inner world of the partner. Each wishes that the other would take in and hold the split-off projections.

Intimacy grows out of partners' increasing ability to understand each other as various levels of encoded messages are sent and received. There is an unstated understanding that when there is communication of deeper aspects of the self, it will be accepted by the other person. Loving relationships are marked by an ability to share things never said before to others. Damage to the relationship occurs as partners refuse, for whatever reason, to accept messages that seem too dangerous, confusing, or unacceptable.

In a marriage that has a flawed holding capacity, communication may serve as a reciprocal barrier against fears of attack, a place to force the other to act out frightening projected feelings, or an entrenched ritualized series of messages that appear to be communications between individuals but more correctly could be described as a script read by two acting as if they were in a relationship. If each uses the other as a receptacle for unconscious archaic pain, a message that the partner is troubled is a signal to "dump."

> SUSAN I work just as hard as you do—how come you don't take me out to dinner?
>
> ROB If you didn't insist that we buy a house this year I wouldn't have

> to work so hard and try to save every cent. Then we could go out
> to dinner.
>
> SUSAN (increasing the stakes) You're the one who wants such an
> expensive house. I just want a place of our own; it doesn't have to
> be that elaborate.
>
> ROB (attacking back) Sure, you can live in some rat-trap. You never
> cared much for taking care of a home or husband. It's always up to
> me to see that we live decently.

Each has said something that triggers a vulnerable area of the other. The couple's communication becomes a series of encoded attack and defense messages, a pattern which has occurred so many times before that the outcome is a foregone conclusion. The emergence of such repetitive patterns exemplifies marital systems and defensive collusions (Dicks, 1967; Willi, 1984), discussed in earlier chapters.

DEFENSIVE COMMUNICATION PATTERNS

Conjoint therapy can run into many snags when the marital relationship is between easily hurt individuals whose defenses include a combination of withdrawal, rage, and shrewd manipulative maneuvers. When a person's early experiences result in an internal mental life largely organized around fantasies of dangerous destructiveness or psychic annihilation, there is an underlying fear that these feelings may emerge to conscious awareness. Rigid verbal defenses are utilized as a protection against disintegration and the pain associated with it. The mind may work exceptionally well, while affect and creativity are repressed in an effort to protect the vulnerable self. The anxiety of the inner world may propel such persons to exceptional achievement while making them difficult to live with (Winnicott, 1986).

Robyn and Jerry

A couple may misperceive each other's needs because their communications are defensive. Here is a typical example of such an interactional pattern:

Robyn and Jerry came into the conjoint therapy session very upset. He was agitated and she had a look of both frustration and resignation.

> JERRY We had a huge fight when we were out driving last weekend.
> The weather was warm; it was such a peaceful day. I was thinking
> how nice things were going and how Robyn was just the way I
> enjoy her. So I told her, "I love you so much." You wouldn't believe

how she acted. It was as though I said something awful instead of something loving.

ROBYN You didn't say "I love you." You said, "I *could* love you so much." Could if what? What do I have to do so you would love me? I never do enough for you. I do 80% of what you ask and you want 100%.

JERRY Why do you always get upset with me? Why do you pick apart what I say? I feel as though you don't want me. There is never a sign of love between us. What you love is the money I make, and you don't want to help me in that.

ROBYN You are always asking me to do things for you every day. Nothing is ever enough. I'm not the one who wants to make a lot of money—you do.

JERRY Before we got married, when I was still trying to convince you, you told me that you like diamonds and furs. You're the one who wants money. And I work my butt off to give it to you.

THERAPIST Jerry, correct me if I'm wrong. It sounds as though you're saying how it feels to you: You work very hard to give Robyn financial security—your way of showing her that you love her—and then she seems unappreciative.

JERRY That's right.

THERAPIST Have you ever checked with her to see what she believes would make her feel loved?

JERRY I think I did. . . . I think I know . . .

THERAPIST Perhaps we should check again now. Robyn, what would let you know you are loved?

ROBYN Jerry knows. I need to be touched and held. I tell him what I need. I've always needed a lot of touching.

JERRY That's what children need, not adults. Robyn was a spoiled brat. She could get anything out of her father. All she had to do was sit on his lap and ask for it.

ROBYN I always felt loved by my father. He held me and touched me and let me sit on his lap. I knew I could have whatever I want. I always knew that. But I never asked for anything. Oh, to stay out an hour later, maybe. I never asked for things. It didn't matter—I knew I was loved. When I try to show Jerry how to make me feel loved, he pushes me away.

JERRY She comes over and tries to climb on my lap. That's infantile. I want a wife, not a baby.

THERAPIST You think Robyn wants material things. You give her a lot financially and you don't know why she is unappreciative and unresponsive. So you think she is spoiled and jaded. You may be giving her what *you* think is important. Even though she helps you with things you ask her to do, it's grudging, withholding. It doesn't seem she is sharing your life joyfully. So you feel unloved. What Robyn says makes her feel loved is the way she got love as a little girl. Robyn, when you come over to give Jerry love it is not as he wants it but as you wish love would be given. You respond, Jerry, by telling her she's infantile. So she withdraws and sulks and says this marriage is not working.

JERRY Well, what do we do?

THERAPIST You might try listening very carefully to what each other wishes for instead of assuming that your own way is the only way to show love.

JERRY You mean, I should treat her like a baby?

THERAPIST Lots of people show love in ways they learned as babies. That's why lovers use baby talk. Love relations are the only place where it is possible to be babied by another person when you're an adult. Robyn can't climb on her father's lap very easily anymore, so she wants to recreate the warm loving feelings with you. That may not be the way you want to be loved. It may even make you uncomfortable. But understand, it is a perfectly legitimate wish even if it's not your way. Perhaps Robyn will be willing to hear from you that when you ask her to come into your business to help, you do it for reasons other than for help in getting things done. You could hire someone for that. What you want is her interest and involvement in what you are doing, something that would show you she cares.

JERRY That's right, that's what I want; but I've sort of given up expecting her to be interested in what I do.

THERAPIST Maybe Robyn needs help to understand what makes you feel loved also.

BUILDING BLOCKS OF COMMUNICATION

While most therapeutic examinations of interpersonal interactions focus on what is expressed verbally, other unofficial but subjectively experienced relatedness is also occurring. The messages are easily recognized in subliminal communications through the body, voice tone, facial expression, and so forth.

As noted in Chapter 4, the developing child relates at several interactional levels at the same time. These are not phase specific but progressive, one domain of relatedness built upon another. Deeply held affects that arose before the infant was capable of symbolization or verbalization are processed differently and expressed through alternative means. As a result, there are simultaneous forms of internal experience: as lived, and as verbally represented. Much that is communicated takes place at an unconscious level. When emotions arise in an intersubjective experience with another, they may be communicated through words or more directly through archaic methods of expression.

While words provide a way to think about affects and emotions and to communicate intersubjectively, language can also create certain problems. Words, for example, permit the communication of two opposing messages — one on a verbal level and another through nonverbal, facial, posturing, and projective expression of affect. However, intersubjective communication is a sharing of affective states, and the development of language may actually make some parts of internal experience less accessible to sharing. With the acquisition of words, it is possible to make decisions about which aspects of inner experience are to be made public and which are to be kept private.

Language is used in a vain attempt to convey clearly important aspects of preverbal internal experience. At best, we are hindered by the lack of enough words and the multiple meanings that can be attributed to words describing affect. When the attempt to convey inner meaning is subsumed by another, there is a great chance that the messages will not be heard or will be translated in incorrect or distorted form. Failure to understand or refusal to respond is the basis for many narcissistic injuries between vulnerable partners. The result is that relationships feel very precarious.

Sometimes clarifying the present in terms of the past makes it easier to understand destructive behavior patterns. A man who recognizes that in his childhood he was intimidated by a domineering, abusive father may use that knowledge either to excuse his continued insecurity around authority figures or to make a decision to change. That a man's mother was consistently late picking him up at school, sometimes forgetting him completely, may explain why he gets so upset when his wife comes home from shopping later than he expected. His rage might bewilder his wife until she understands the source of his feelings of abandonment — the hurt child standing alone at a curbside. Her wish not to have to live according to his experience of time may look to him like a wish to hurt him until he realizes that her actions are part of her own search for autonomy. Each needs help in understanding what the other is communicating.

A woman in treatment acknowledged that she desperately wants a loving relationship but avoids men because she fears the anger that she anticipates will occur. Recognition that she was intimidated by her over-bearing father may clarify her current feelings for her lover without chang-ing either those feelings or her behavior. Additional steps are necessary to recognize whether messages are direct or encoded unconscious ones, and what triggers their reemergence in the present relationship, in order to develop new, less threatening ways of interacting.

To differ in relationships is not unusual. To think the other is wrong or bad for seeing things differently or disagreeing lays the groundwork for narcissistic injury even in a relatively caring relationship. When a marriage is made up of persons who are prone to experiences of narcissistic injury, it is crucial for therapeutic treatment of the couple to take into account the fragile, easily damaged self of each one. The couple's arguments often reflect their joint tendency to defend against humiliation and fragmenta-tion, especially when either or both has disavowed important needs and views aspects of the self as illegitimate or unacceptable.

As one listens to communications, it is possible, by examining the contextual framework, to determine whether a given utterance is meant to convey a single meaning or several. How does the message fit in with previous and subsequent messages? Are the messages given in the words, the voice, and the bodily movements in synchrony or in conflict? Does there appear to be an effort to provoke another into feeling upset or reactive? Is there some triggering factor for one or both that causes the defensive encoding of messages? It is especially important to keep in mind that an utterance or action that triggers disturbing feelings in another may be an attempt to project toxic or frightening affect away from the self.

DECODING DISTORTED COMMUNICATION

The primary advantage and the primary difficulty of doing therapy in a marital context are one and the same: The therapist can observe the dis-turbed communications as they are occurring. The difficulty is that the interaction between husband and wife can become so intense that the therapist feels things will soon be out of control. With patients who are prone to collusive interactions, highly emotional transactions must be translated from the language of affects to the language of feelings. Con-scious understanding must be included in the transactions. This is why the responses of each, for a time, must go through a decoding process by the therapist. "What was said," "what was meant," "what else was implied, but unsaid," "correct me when I translate your meaning incorrectly," are said by the therapist in alternating responses to each partner.

In order to decode messages appropriately and safely in a way that reduces or eliminates damaging interactional patterns, care must be taken to avoid recreating the feeling that caused the defenses to arise initially. Once empathically exposed and contained, feelings generate responsive messages that reflect improved coping capacities. However, in spite of one's recognition of the need to hear and accept the underlying messages, therapeutic listening and decoding are not easy, since the messages the therapist must translate are defensively encoded because they are so painful.

When therapists encourage spouses to communicate with each other, it is important to recognize that the word "communicate," like the word "love," has many meanings. We have seen how miscommunication occurs. Preconscious experience and unconscious affect are out of the realm of awareness. In individual or conjoint treatment, when the correct words are identified for a heretofore "unthought known" (Bollas, 1987), there is a great sense of relief. In fact, it is crucial to train spouses to "hear" each other at levels other than simply the conscious verbal one.

A therapist must make a decision about when to translate underlying messages and when to try to help the partners translate. A lot depends upon how much experience the therapist has with a particular couple and upon how much the partners have learned to trust the therapy as a container of hurt or guilty feelings. In conjoint treatment a therapist's metacommunicative comments on the nature of the relationship often alternate with empathic responses about underlying feelings. For example, as a couple negotiates how they will manage career and household arrangements to meet the needs of both, a single comment by the husband betrays several levels of communication. The wife may respond to the husband at any of these levels.

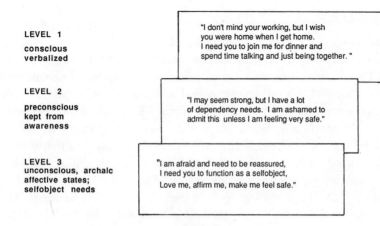

LEVEL 1

conscious
verbalized

"I don't mind your working, but I wish you were home when I get home. I need you to join me for dinner and spend time talking and just being together. "

LEVEL 2

preconscious
kept from
awareness

"I may seem strong, but I have a lot of dependency needs. I am ashamed to admit this unless I am feeling very safe."

LEVEL 3
unconscious, archaic
affective states;
selfobject needs

"I am afraid and need to be reassured, I need you to function as a selfobject, Love me, affirm me, make me feel safe."

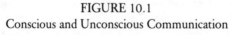

FIGURE 10.1
Conscious and Unconscious Communication

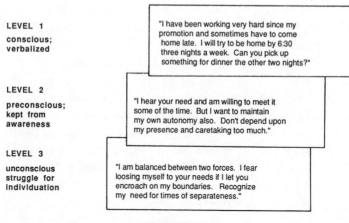

LEVEL 1

conscious;
verbalized

"I have been working very hard since my promotion and sometimes have to come home late. I will try to be home by 6:30 three nights a week. Can you pick up something for dinner the other two nights?"

LEVEL 2

preconscious;
kept from
awareness

"I hear your need and am willing to meet it some of the time. But I want to maintain my own autonomy also. Don't depend upon my presence and caretaking too much."

LEVEL 3

unconscious
struggle for
individuation

"I am balanced between two forces. I fear loosing myself to your needs if I let you encroach on my boundaries. Recognize my need for times of separateness."

FIGURE 10.2
Conscious and Unconscious Communication

The husband's comment on the surface is simple. But it is easy to see from his expression, tone of voice, posture, and ultimately, his conscious admission, that there are several messages underneath his overt verbalization. Figure 10.1 shows three levels of communication by the husband.

The wife makes a predictable and reasonable response on the surface, but it also contains layers of covert communication, as seen in Figure 10.2.

Rick and Ellie

The following is a conversation between Rick and Ellie, a young couple who lived together for two years and have been married for one and a half years. They have been on the verge of separation almost since the time they married. Ellie says that she never expected to feel so stifled in the marriage and often wonders aloud if she made a mistake. Rick has tried desperately to make the relationship work. He is a clean-cut young man who looks considerably younger than his 32 years. When they came into therapy he said that he took a long time to marry and, because of his religious beliefs, considers marriage a permanent commitment. The more Ellie questions the relationship, the more anxious he becomes. As his anxiety increases, he tries to find ways to hold onto the relationship more tightly. Ellie feels constricted and wants to pull away. The nonverbal interpretations are based upon my inferences and upon knowledge I gained in the course of conjoint therapy with this couple.

The top layer of each communication is rational, verbal, and interactive. The second reflects the nonverbal areas of the psyche which developed in the first years of life. The third goes to the deepest and earliest beginnings of the individual when the self of the child was emerging as separate and yet dependent.

RICK ──────────▶ ELLIE

1. "Last night when we made love I felt that you really wanted this relationship to work. I felt at peace." (verbal message)
2. "I seek a feeling of merger with you to provide me with a feeling of wholeness." (nonverbal and unconscious)
3. "Without you near me I fear psychic disintegration." (deeply unconscious message of archaic terror)

ELLIE ──────────▶ RICK

1. "Last night was good but you would like to believe that our problems are now over." (verbally stated)
2. "There is something very wrong in this relationship for me." (conscious, nonverbalized)
3. "When we are too close, I feel engulfed by you and want to get out of here before there is nothing left of me." (unconscious response to husband's archaic merger fantasy and fear of loss of self.)

RICK ──────────▶ ELLIE

1. "I try to do things that will make you be with me in a warm affirming manner." (conscious, sometimes verbally stated in attempt to plan time together)
2. "I am afraid that you will leave me if I don't work hard to hold onto you." (fear of abandonment)
3. "Without you near I fear chaos, a fragmented self." (archaic fear of loss of cohesion; if affect emerges anxiety is compounded by shame)

ELLIE ──────────▶ RICK

1. "I want to be able to make my own plans and see my friends without your getting angry at me." (verbalized)
2. "When you get too close, there is no room for me to breathe." (preconscious, known but not specifically put into words)

3. "This relationship feels devouring to me." (unconscious affective anxiety)

Ellie gave the same messages to Rick on many occasions. Her verbal messages were different but the underlying feelings were the same. Rick understood her wish to distance herself from him but, rather than recognizing her fears, was preoccupied with his own. He increasingly tried to hold her near to him. The more she felt him "clutching" at her, the more she found ways to be distant.

ELLIE ————————▶ RICK

1. Verbal messages:
   a. "How about taking separate vacations this year?"
   b. "I need to have my own friends."
   c. "Please don't call me at work so often."
2. Conscious but nonstated message:
   a. "I feel less and less and less involved in this relationship."
   b. "I will distance myself from you."
   c. "I need a space for myself."
3. Thoughts that are at the preconscious or unconscious level:
   a. "I want your love, but not your version of closeness."
   b. "I intend to maintain myself as a separate person."
   c. "I must protect my own boundaries or I will lose myself and become a part of you."

Other times, when Ellie said things with no underlying distancing messages, Rick read into them what he expected to hear. When Rick finished law school the year that they married, Ellie said that it was now her turn to go back to school. Rick, knowing how time-consuming it had been to study, interpreted Ellie's wish as another way to distance herself from him. He resisted her efforts in a number of ways, causing Ellie to confirm her impressions of the marriage as confining and intolerable to her. Once a partner comes to expect an underlying message from past communications, a communication that gives a straight message can easily be read as though it is part of the previously recognized pattern.

The therapist draws on several forms of evidence in listening for clues to the content of the partners' messages to one another: (1) the words and actions of either partner; (2) awareness of the nature of the relational space between the mates, as when a seemingly innocuous remark is received with great emotion, a welling up of tears, anger, etc.; and (3) the therapist's own

internal reaction toward one of the mates or both—the immediate experience within the consulting room as well as the wishes or fantasies about the
spouses that remain with the therapist after they have left. In the next
chapter the last element will be discussed in further detail.

It is important for the marital therapist to listen to each partner, allowing
communication to proceed as long as the partners are hearing and responding to each other in nondestructive ways. As soon as there is a reaction that
either appears to be part of a collusive pattern or presents messages that
conflict with what was said earlier, the therapist points out the discrepancy
with a request for clarification and assistance from both. When the message
sent by one partner seems quite different from the message heard by the
other, it is time for some decoding on the part of the therapist. By observing the empathic communication being modeled in the course of such
decoding, which includes sensing and responding to nonverbal messages,
partners learn that they do not need to act on feelings of being attacked.
They have permission to respond "it hurts me when you say that," rather
than sending back escalating cutting remarks.

The goal is a microcommunication of the interaction process, an examination of the relationship between the intrapsychic and the interpersonal,
and the opening of new paths to modification. This requires a focus on the
process rather than on the content of the encounter. By taking the time
during the session to stop at times of heightened affectivity and to consciously focus with the partners on the minute details of feelings as they
emerge, the therapist can interrupt the cycle of injury and fear.

EXPANDING THE LISTENING PROCESS

At the beginning of treatment, partners who are narcissistically vulnerable
are not asked to paraphrase what they heard each other say, because failure
to read a message correctly raises feelings of embarrassment and anxiety in
one partner or both. Putting them on the spot raises their defenses and
creates a threatening situation. Both members of the couple are more likely
to become engaged if, at the beginning, the therapist acts as the conduit for
communication. That is, she or he repeats the partners' messages in a clear,
calm, accepting tone, which, in addition to supporting communication, has
the highly desirable effect of modeling the prescribed procedure for the
partners.

As the therapist repeats and paraphrases, he or she watches for nonverbal
cues that the sender has been injured by the comments. If there is no sign of
agreement, no body language that signals feeling understood, it is necessary
to check with the sender, saying, "I may have missed something. Please tell

me more so I will understand, or please correct me." After a paraphrase that meets with a nod or verbalized agreement, the other partner is enlisted and asked for any comments. The message is treated as though it came clearly and directly from the other. As time goes on, the speaker pauses for corroboration and the receiver responds automatically. The therapist is careful to speak to both mates, alternating or at the same time. Even when only one has been speaking, both are included in the therapeutic response. All comments to either or both are really interventions aimed at both.

An obvious way to improve communication is to teach couples to pay attention to each other's nonverbal messages, to body language, facial expressions, signs of tension, and so on. Another skill that can be taught is how to become aware of one's internal process as the receiver of various, sometimes mixed messages, in the context of the interaction. Either party in the communicative exchange can add a dimension of understanding by tuning in to his or her own experience and decoding the transmission for multilevel meaning.

Of course, even if partners understand each other, they can launch damaging miscommunications. On the other hand, spouses who know each other's emotional languages can communicate well even when they disagree. Many couples develop listening processes that allow each to explain his or her own subjective truth without feeling invalidated or undermined. Where there are narcissistic vulnerabilities, but no history of injury to each other, occasional failures of empathy or differing views do not cause defense-attack patterns to come into play. What such couples know intuitively or learned in their families of origin are skills that can be taught to others.

For the narcissistically vulnerable person who is used to a very different response and expects hurts in current relationships to be as damaging as past injuries, special care must be taken to encourage a feeling of safety in the presence of an intimate partner. They must not only learn a new way of communicating but also acquire increasing tolerance for the unintentional mistakes of others. When there is great need for others and yet exquisite sensitivity to responses that may damage, the therapist must be skilled in finding ways to communicate affective experiences occurring in the relational space between the mates.

CHANGING PATTERNS OF COMMUNICATION

Difficulties around communication in the relational space between partners arise not only from the problems presented, but also from underlying issues — power and powerlessness, love and hate, dependency and autonomy. Treatment of a couple may include problem-solving, methods of modifying behaviors, and ways of restructuring family dynamics. Therapy must also recognize humiliation, aggression, and sexuality—unknown, unstated, and unacceptable factors. It is difficult to make long-term changes in interactions between partners without helping them understand and modify the ways that they use their relationship to express their individual emotions.

Therapy allows the mates to examine their expectations, fears and hurts in terms of current reality and past experiences. It then becomes possible to see how values incorporated from the family of origin are causing frustrating interactions. As partners come to understand each other's requests and behavior, they reexamine their own expectations and often begin to understand that the other's behavior is based on old wounds, not simply on a wish to blame or attack the present mate. It is possible to negotiate a modification in their behavior that will allow for a new, more realistic marital contract.

Communication is oriented toward restructuring marital interactions by systematically investigating and clarifying the transference distortions. In the attempt to understand, it begins to become clear to both that projected feelings and actions of each one result in intense hurts and defensive actions by the other. Sometimes their actions are designed to do this, either as a way of defending against hurt or as retribution. At other times, although there was no intention to hurt the other, when either one experiences a hurt it is assumed that the other inflicted it purposely. At these times a neutral observer who serves as decoder and translator of communication can really make a difference. Once the therapeutic sessions are transformed into a safe haven for the mates to experience what is going on at a deeper level between them, it is possible to stop the session when either one looks upset or hurt or when the response sounds suspiciously like a defense against something.

The process of understanding and absorbing the messages, allowing oneself to be a receptive container, and attempting to understand what triggered the reaction at this particular moment provides a space in which inner problems can begin to be examined and managed. Pieces of the interactional process may be frozen to create a "time out" in which the exact words, feeling states of each, and defense-counterdefense patterns can be studied nonjudgmentally. If defenses are looked at in terms of what they might be defending against rather than in terms of how inappropriate they are to the current relationship, it is possible to return repeatedly and safely to the reasons for the defense.

Taking time to stop and examine the messages that couples send and receive at the surface level and at a deeper level often gives the partners new insight into each other. Sometimes there is a discrimination between inner representational images and the apparent reality of the spouse's personality. Partners are generally relieved to learn that a mate's behavior and statements are not meant as an attack but as a way of protecting against hurt. They are encouraged to talk about their hurt and disappointment instead of continuing a cycle of blame. Each is helped to communicate better by overt verbal repetition of their own thoughts and feelings. Such repetition, which reinforces reflection on the message, is carried out in a modulated tone of acceptance and with explanation of the reasons for the statements. If the therapist does not understand what is being communicated or is confused by conflicting messages, the interaction may be stopped with a request for clarification. Partners soon learn that confusion comes out of the sender's obscure communication and/or the listener's difficulty in receiving. In either case there are valid reasons, if time is taken to explore them. These are to be seen as "no fault" communication lapses: The "sending" partner has a chance to clarify the message; the "receiver" can ask for clarification and ask again if the meaning of the message remains unclear. The relationship between past and present may explain what seems confusing in the communication process.

Some key phrases for acting as a conduit are, "What occurs to me . . ." "I have a hunch about something," and, "A thought came into my mind as you were speaking." Putting statements into this sort of frame dispels the appearance that the therapist is the carrier of truth, the decider of right and wrong, or the judge of what should be done. No one knows for sure why another person reacts in a particular, seemingly unreasonable manner. Only by conveying an effort to understand and asking for each person's more knowing assistance in determining what is going on internally can the therapist engage in a working alliance with each partner. Particularly in conjoint sessions, the therapist must be careful to avoid the appearance of knowing who is right, thus putting one mate or the other on the spot or raising feelings of shame or humiliation.

A main purpose of such supported dialogues is the revision of negative attributions on the part of each partner into statements of needs, vulnerabilities, and concerns. What might have been seen as negative is instead looked at in a positive light. Symptoms are identified as attempts at finding a resolution to a joint problem. With this awareness, couples may be able to change patterns of defense and retaliation. As understanding increases and defenses are reduced, the two may come to be remarkably responsive to each other.

TRANSMUTATION AND TRANSFORMATION

Slowly, what had been out of the realm of conscious awareness begins to emerge. That does not mean that there will be no hurt. However, the hurts and injuries that take place during the course of such a mutual investigation of patterns in an intimate relationship allow for a certain transmuting internalization (Kohut, 1977), or transformation of internal structures. Each partner's tolerance for some degree of future psychic injury builds up. Through acquisition of new information and through the experience of modeling, a partner who is motivated toward improving a relationship has new tools to use in the follow-up at home.

Lasting change in marital therapy requires a repeated focus on the latent messages in communication. In that way, feelings and fantasies that are only dimly perceived or not perceived consciously at all, but that profoundly affect all interactions, can be acknowledged and confronted in therapy. By observing how individuals interact and communicate with one another and with the therapist, it is possible to define the important problems at issue for that couple and the aspects that trigger vulnerability and defensive patterns.

It is necessary for both partners to examine their needs at moments of anxiety or hurt, their feelings of grief and loss, their wishes for praise and approval. Listening to the therapist respond with empathy to the vulnerability and pain that lie below what appears to be a demand or attack will eventually make partners aware of their areas of sensitivity and the feelings of helplessness arising from unmet needs. The therapist helps the couple to reinterpret anger, to recognize that rage may be based upon an inability to assert needs and demands so they can be met. Each partner must be allowed, as much as possible, to express needs freely in a nonjudgmental, empathic atmosphere. Each partner learns to hear the needs of the other, hidden behind demands and rage.

Spouses become more responsive to each other because they have been observing the therapist's empathic listening and learning methods for giving and receiving responses to previously submerged, frightening feelings. They learn how to hear messages that usually are sent only in encoded form. As these messages are received and accepted, new communications may be sent in less guarded form. As it becomes less necessary to mobilize defenses against old needs and feelings, a transformation often occurs. Narcissistic demandingness can be replaced by an even, consistent assertiveness; the timidity and withdrawal once needed to protect against shame and embarrassment are replaced by a willingness to expose high aspirations and deep devotion.

By the time communication patterns have been clarified, much work has been done in conjoint sessions. Often the marriage has been stabilized. Both partners have learned how their misinterpretations of each other tend to set up confirmatory interactions. They are encouraged to use what they have learned and what they have seen the therapist do to resolve interactional issues between them.

CHAPTER 11

The Therapist's Empathic Self as a Tool of Treatment

In this chapter I will focus on the therapist's self as an instrument for the effective treatment of couples. I am convinced that the therapist is the most important factor in successful psychodynamic treatment of relationship problems. The person of the therapist includes professional training and experience, but the social and cultural background, family-of-origin dynamics, and personal developmental history of the therapist are also essential factors in the course of treatment. Furthermore, I contend that a lack of a well-fitting match between patient and therapist is a primary factor in many therapeutic failures.

Therapists, it must be noted, are imperfect mortals, as are we all, and have come through very similar processes of learning to be in the world as have most patients. It is, in fact, this very commonality of flawed humanity that makes it possible to respond empathically to the dilemmas presented by our patients. Not only who we are but how we have learned to use ourselves, our resources, and our internal awareness provide the benefits to those with whom we work therapeutically.

I begin this final chapter of the book, therefore, with a short review of the significant issues that influence intimate relationships, and that may influence the values and personality of the therapist and the choice of therapy as a profession. I then consider the ways that a therapist who is trained in the listening process may come to understand the many voices of the unconscious that are present in every therapeutic experience. I will touch on topics that concern all therapists, such as empathy as a tool of treatment, the dyadic nature of transference and countertransference, the use of projective identification and projective counter-identification as a tuning fork for receiving the meaning of messages, and the therapist's emotional response to the couple and to each of the mates.

THE CHOICE OF THERAPY AS A PROFESSION

Early interactional sequences become entrenched prototypes for later intimate and family relationships. Once a way of being in the world is ingrained, it operates without conscious awareness and is the motivator of a wide range of behaviors. Choice of a mate and choice of a career may be determined by these unconscious factors. Reactions to closeness and distance, power and submissiveness, love, hate and indifference, happiness and grief, sickness and health, work and play are all influenced by early interactional programming.

A person's choice of vocation brings into focus much of his developmental dynamics as well as many unconscious forces influencing his life. Miller has described parentified persons who "not only become mothers, confidants, comforters, advisors, supporters to their own mothers, but also take over the responsibility for their siblings and eventually develop a special sensitivity to unconscious signals manifesting the needs of others" (1981, p. 9). A selective factor in choosing psychotherapy as a career may be a need to relate more intimately to others, to understand oneself better, to repeat a pattern of caretaking that began in childhood, to resolve personal problems, or to meet needs for power, admiration, "love." Psychotherapy is a relatively "safe" way of relating in an intimate way with others. In fact, the choice of a career in psychotherapy may represent a way of solving the therapist's personal problems. It would appear that some children who are unable to get their own nascent needs met and are required to take a parental role early under threat of being isolated from meaningful ties with people (Boszormenyi-Nagy and Krasner, 1986) are in danger of growing up to become therapists.

COUNTERTRANSFERENCE AND THERAPEUTIC NEUTRALITY

The tensions that emerge in conjoint treatment of couples or families may be at once voyeuristic and overwhelming (Brown, 1984). The therapist moves into the most intimate relationship between husband and wife or father and mother, and may not know a way of resolving certain issues. The wish to take charge and make the situation manageable may result in focusing on aspects that can be resolved, while putting aside those issues that stir up too many memories and emotions within the therapist.

Marital work, even more than individual treatment, seems to be influenced by countertransference reactions of the therapist. However, I have rarely heard therapists acknowledge that their own personal views have any bearing on whether or not couples with whom they work stay together, separate, or divorce. The therapeutic stance of many is that when they see a couple, they will do what is best for the two individuals involved. Each partner, feel such therapists, must decide to do what is best for his or her personal development. That statement, in itself, betrays a common value in our current culture.

There are many reports of therapists who felt that the mental health of one person was being damaged by the other. The question arises, "What keeps this person in such a destructive relationship?" It is all too easy to assume that it is only pathology that holds the collusive bonds of the marriage together. Successful treatment could then easily lead to termination of the marriage.

If the therapeutic intervention is not deemed helpful by one of the mates or if the marriage appears to deteriorate during the course of treatment, it is not unusual for the therapist to end up working with one or the other individual in treatment. I have known therapists who have helped one of the partners "to get strong enough to get a divorce." This may leave the partner who does not want a divorce with neither therapist nor spouse.

Therapeutic neutrality assumes that the therapist should have no judgments about the relationship. This, too, may be an inappropriate stance— or even a negative one—in the context of conjoint therapy. Many couples fear that if their real feelings come through, their relationship will unravel or end explosively. They fear abandonment or attack or both. At the same time, there is likely to be considerable ambivalence about a distressing, unhappy interaction. If both of them fear the disintegration of the relationship, and if the therapist has made it clear that the decision to stay married or to separate is in their hands, they might feel a pressure to hold back dangerous feelings. The safety of therapy is, thereby, disturbed. Frightening feelings can only come out in a safe atmosphere—a containing environment.

THE EFFECT OF THE THERAPIST'S LIFE SITUATION ON TREATMENT

All adults have made decisions about relationships: to get married or stay single, to stay married or get a divorce. The decisions a therapist has made about his or her own life are likely to affect the reactions to those who are dealing with similar issues. The therapist who has decided to leave what feels like an intolerable marital situation may think in those terms when he or she sees a similarly unhappy situation in a patient's life. Although a therapist's personal history is not shared with patients, thoughts, affects and attitudes, are communicated in many ways other than verbally. In this aspect, care must be taken to avoid a countertransference problem.

Once a therapeutic alliance has been established, many people, particularly those with narcissistic vulnerabilities, tend to idealize and overidentify with the conscious and unconscious values of the helping person. There is a tendency to trust the ideas of the therapist and a wish to act in ways that will meet with the approval of the therapist.

Whether the life choice of the therapist involved leaving a difficult marriage or staying in an equally difficult one, that personal decision is bound to affect feelings about the appropriateness of marital separation. I have had a number of patients who recalled that a previous therapist, after seeing them one or several times, suggested that they consider divorce as an alternative. As one frustrated husband told me, "I didn't have to go to a therapist for that; I thought of that myself lots of times."

One therapist with a great deal of experience described the changing awareness in her attitude toward relationships over the years. In the late 1960s a patient came in with a copy of Betty Friedan's *The Feminine Mystique*, complaining that it was a description of her life. The patient described herself as "living an unproductive life, in an unfulfilling marriage, and needing more personal growth." The therapist felt very much "in synch" with her patient. They worked together for almost two years, during which time she assisted the patient through a divorce, a return to school, and a growing feeling of power and determination. Recently the therapist received a card from her ex-patient announcing her new position as a real estate broker. The announcement brought up many issues for the therapist. Almost 20 years had passed since they terminated treatment. In the interim the therapist had divorced, moved to Europe for several years, and was now back in the United States, living alone. She has had many experiences that she might not have had if she had remained in her own marriage. But, she added, she has not achieved the greater personal fulfillment that she sought. She is no longer so sure that divorce is the answer to problems in relationships. She wonders whether her ideal of personal growth was actually accomplished, or whether she just exchanged one set of problems for another. In retrospect she wonders if her work with this patient would have been the same had she known then what she knows now. What she does recognize is that her perspective on love, life, and marriage has changed considerably in the intervening years, and that her encouragement of individual growth at the cost of a relationship would not be given so freely today. Would the course of treatment and the outcome have differed if her responses had been different? Perhaps not. There is no way to be certain.

At times, when the values and principles of the therapist are in conflict with those of one of the mates, it is difficult to correctly hear and empathically respond to what that person may be experiencing. Our impartial lenses may be distorted by a value-laden prejudice. Beliefs about homosexuality, affairs, or racial differences, for example, may bias the listening stance; messages are then misconstrued. As we work with patients, our values, beliefs and personal history have great impact on the treatment. Therapists convey the mores of our culture. We are not neutral. We have our own life experiences—our own marriage, relationship, and sexual issues. Tolerance of different ways of thinking and acting varies widely.

At other times, emotional expectations cannot be negotiated. For instance, a Middle Eastern couple came into treatment over the husband's demand that his wife "obey him" in all things. "If I wanted equality I would have married an American girl," he adamantly said. My immediate negative reaction had to be put aside so that I could hear their marital contract. The wife did not disagree with his values or want to change them. Her complaint was that, if she was to spend most evenings and weekends with his family, she wanted both permission to see more of her family during the day and an agreement by him occasionally to attend her family gatherings. When he refused she considered a separation. He brought her to therapy so that I could straighten her out—a difficult task indeed from my viewpoint. During the course of our work together, I presented my reservations and said that I wondered why a man with his cultural background and his view of women would seek out a woman therapist. "She will listen to you," he said. I wondered at the time if he thought that I had no opinion on the subject, or if he thought that I agreed with him. After several months in treatment, it became clear to me that he had transferred to me his feelings toward his mother. He took my neutral stance as confirmation that I was there to take care of his needs and that I would encourage his wife to do as he wished. They are still married. I cannot imagine how she puts up with his demands.

In a class on psychodynamic marital therapy a therapist described her treatment of a man who was heavily involved in a secret affair with a younger woman and thinking of leaving his wife of 25 years. There was a wide variation in reaction among members of the class. While the class proceeded to make some assessment of the man's individual dynamics and underlying problems based upon the present material, several women reacted negatively and had difficulty even discussing the underlying dynamics of this man. As we examined the reactions of various members of the class, it became clear that the situation hit close to home for some, particularly a few who had somewhat precarious relationships themselves. "Could it happen to me?" was a question that interfered with the attempt to understand the issues of this patient. Could they work with such a situation? Most said that this would not affect their treatment if this were a patient in treatment. I could only advise that when personal issues become intermingled with treatment it is time for consultation with another therapist.

When the therapist's emotional reactions to the couple or the issues presented are very strong, therapy often fails. Immersion into the treatment causes a loss of boundaries, along with a loss of ability to cognitively decode and contain the intensely swirling emotional reactions that emerge. The explanation generally given is that these are "difficult" or "resistant" patients. But those who seek help are looking for some way to deal with issues that they cannot contain within themselves. It is the role of the therapist to develop ways of dealing with emotional containment, boundary issues, and difficult interpersonal reactions, by using the tools within.

Jack and Linda

Recently I saw a couple, Jack and Linda, who presented me with a dilemma of values. After struggling to attain empathy, I was relieved when our sessions terminated after two months.

Jack and Linda separated after 12 years together, 10 of them as a married couple. For the past eight years they have functioned as a team, acting, writing, and directing for a major film studio. One month ago they separated, supposedly at Linda's insistence. She was increasingly upset by what she considered Jack's lack of reciprocal support and even betrayal in some of their joint projects. When she left their home, she said that a short period of time apart might help her clear her mind, and that she hoped they would soon reunite. The following day Linda said that she was miserable and wanted to return home. Jack told her that he did not want her back yet and that they should remain separated for a while. A few days later he had a young woman move into the house that he and Linda had shared together.

When, upon entering marital therapy, they were asked what each of them hoped to accomplish, Linda said that she wanted to resolve whatever had been going wrong in their relationship and come back together. Jack said that he was not ready for that, and yet there was so much good in their relationship that he did not want to give it up. He intended to maintain his relationship with his lover and at the same time continue to work professionally with Linda. They worked together extraordinarily well, he explained. Linda said that, if he was talking about continuing to live with his new girlfriend and convert their own relationship into a purely professional partnership, she was not ready to work toward that. They would have to end their marriage and then give it some time. She added that the situation made her very angry. She worked hard to help him achieve so much professionally. Now he made a big income and was very successful, but she would have to start all over.

I wondered how I could help them, inasmuch as his actions and expectations were so against my own principles. There was no way that I could put aside my feelings and agree that Jack's decision to replace Linda while continuing to benefit from her professional support was morally acceptable. Yet, both wanted to work on the relationship, professing to have widely different goals.

In the two months that we worked together I found that I was trying to help Linda deal with what she saw as the demanding, inconsiderate, and immoral attitude of her husband. He remained calm as she raged at him. Then, angry at him and at me for not repairing their relationship, she terminated treatment.

At the time I fully understood her reaction to his behavior. It was not until long afterward that I began to reexamine my focus with this couple. What was making it so hard for Jack to live with Linda? What had he put up with before acting-out in this inappropriate manner? If he really cared for her and wished to maintain a relationship, why didn't he ask his girlfriend to move out and try to work on the marriage? How bad had it been for him? I now wondered whether the cutting anger that I saw in therapeutic sessions was a reaction to his behavior, or whether it had always been there as part of the relationship. Was his nonresponsiveness because of his guilt, or was his role in the marriage to stay calm while she was free to become enraged?

I do not know the answers to these questions. I wasn't able to investigate these issues at the time because my emotions were interfering with my thinking. My interest was directed by a conviction that his behavior was causing the problem. My values made it difficult to empathize with the pain that he might have experienced in the 12 years that they were together.

THE THERAPIST'S EMOTIONAL RESPONSE TO THE COUPLE

Couples generally seek help at the point where the situation feels untenable and they are close to hopeless. The system is in the process of breaking down and they are particularly vulnerable. Despite any attempt to the contrary, the therapist cannot work with a marital or family system without becoming in some ways immersed in it. It is necessary to use the permeability of the system's boundaries in ways that promote the relationship and allow destructive aspects to emerge and be dealt with. The attempt at an empathic, absolutely evenhanded response is a necessary condition of treatment of the narcissistically vulnerable marriage.

Sometimes this is difficult. With some couples therapists will feel a distance, boredom broken by periods of interest, but no life. It is at these times when I may acknowledge, to myself first, that some direct messages are being passed between the unconscious of one or both of them and my own. I ask myself if they are trying to share with me some helplessness within or if they fear that I will be threatened by the intensity of their inner experience. Perhaps they are deathly afraid of any real emotion. It is difficult to live in a relationship with another if terror arises every time emotions do. No wonder they are locked in a battle for control, pleading with each other to accede to any demand. The alternative is too frightening.

Some challenging behavior is a highly active unconscious endeavor designed to make others experience the relationship in a particular way. Some spouses use each other as a vehicle for containment of emotions that are felt to be intrinsically dangerous and intolerable.

Stuart and Zelda

Stuart and Zelda had been married for 16 years when Zelda entered therapy depressed and unable to cope with her marital problems. She said repeatedly in the initial session that she could not describe her husband and that the therapist would have to meet him to understand. She went on to say that she had always believed that her level-headed stability would enable her to handle her husband's highs and lows. Stuart was an exciting man who was never able to settle down with what he had. He always reached out for more, and so far, "his schemes had mostly worked," she said. He had bought a house "over his head," then found an even bigger one, built a business "on the come" from nothing, and always had excitement surrounding them. She never knew what to expect next. She recognized that there was something quite manic in their lifestyle, but before she always knew that she could contain his excesses. Now it was becoming too much.

In the past he had allowed her to place limits on his activities. But lately neither he nor his wife could contain his acquisitive activities. He had to have everything he wanted, instantly. And he became intensely agitated when he felt that he was deprived. A few weeks before, he had decided that they must make an addition to their home to house an art gallery for pictures that he had recently purchased. The house had been completely redone the year before when they bought it. There was not enough money because he had been buying art at a frantic pace. She went over their accounts with him and told him that he must stop spending, they were going broke. One morning a bulldozer came and broke through their kitchen wall. "That was it," she said. She decided either she must take the children and leave or they must enter marital therapy.

It was clear upon meeting Stuart that his wife's consternation was well-founded. He explained his need to have Zelda near him all the time—with him "joyfully." Seeing her upset made him feel as if he had done something bad. He came into therapy with her so she would stop being upset. "You don't know how much I hold myself back when I want things," he added. In an effort to not overburden her, he explained, he worked hard to have many people and many things in his life. He had been afraid that he would wear Zelda out with his enormous needs. In the end, though, both she and their bank account had become depleted. As hard as he tried, he could not stop himself in his effort to ward off depression and fill the emptiness within.

Stuart's internal dilemma took up a great deal of his energy and was acted out in manic activity—building, buying, and developing new ideas. Underlying his problem was an inability to reconcile his loving and destructive feelings. He had old, unresolved angry reactions toward his parents for their failure to give him what he needed as a child. He appeared as a success in the world and a failure in relationships, with his wife, his children, and his parents. His home was the biggest, the best, and the most secure; his inner life the most threatening and empty.

He loved the thrill of business, the "war games" and the ultimate submission of both colleagues and competitors. Never would he be the impotent, humiliated victim of more powerful aggressive figures. He would protect himself and his family from becoming victimized at all costs. "The world is not a safe place," he said, convinced that the threat was external rather than coming from within himself. Pursuing the wish to protect those whom he loved from danger, he could never stop achieving.

Therapy with this couple often felt like a rollercoaster. At times he was euphoric and she was depressed. Other times they both seemed to stabilize and I thought treatment was progressing well, only to find chaos reemerging within a few weeks. I found myself feeling frustrated and inadequate, a sure sign of my failure to contain unexpressed needs, fears, and aggression. At one point, Zelda left, thus confirming his belief that ultimately he was alone and had to protect himself from the dangerous world outside.

When Zelda called to cancel the marital therapy after she had left Stuart, she said it was a relief to go home at night without the "craziness." I told her that I understood—and I truly did. I, too, felt a sense of relief that we were stopping.

After a few weeks Zelda called and said that she had very much missed the excitement that Stuart brought to the relationship; she had become even more depressed during their separation. They were together again and wanted to resume treatment.

It was not with great anticipation that I scheduled a session. At this point, however, they acknowledged that we were dealing with more than a marital problem. Stuart accepted referral for individual treatment with a therapist who specialized in psychopharmacology. The mood swings receded, and marital work became possible again.

It was interesting to observe the systemic change that took place as medication helped Stuart to function more calmly. Zelda's underlying issues, including phobias and depression, emerged. She too entered individual therapy. Their unconscious collusion of mutually reciprocal protection against underlying pathology had broken down. True change became possible as our work progressed.

TOOLS OF THE THERAPIST: COUNTERTRANSFERENCE AND EMPATHY

Among the least understood of the psychodynamic processes are the ways that human beings develop the ability to comprehend the internal experience of another. The psychoanalytic literature and the family systems literature contain numerous descriptions of the many ways in which closely related people use one another to carry and act out pathology. In severe pathology, the patient's history often reveals a borderline or psychotic parent whose mixed messages caused chaos and confusion in the lives of those who were involved intimately with him or her. The undifferentiated family ego mass (Bowen, 1978) and the inability to achieve individuation (Mahler, Pine, and Bergman, 1975) are indicators of how emotional reactivity may be transferred from one member in an intimate relationship to another.

The same complex processes that begin as "involuntary affective experiences" (Basch, 1983) later become transformed into bodily sensations and behavioral responses. Emotional reactions characteristic of parent-child and analyst-patient dyads also occur in the marital relationship. Through a process of empathic understanding of the unconscious or undeclared processes between husband and wife, the therapist can help mates translate covertly transmitted messages. The partners are assisted in sharing with each other the underlying affects and defenses that each has felt necessary for self-preservation within the relationship.

The goal is to offer an environment that will enhance empathic understanding between the mates (see Chapter 9) and to model for them a method of listening at a deeper level (see Chapter 10). This difficult task requires a willingness to make space for "the arrival of news from within the self" (Bollas, 1987, p. 239). When the mind is receptive, it becomes possible to attune oneself to the relational space in the therapeutic setting. Projections, introjections, and projective identifications are met with an empathic stance, as part of an investigation of the internal state of the partners, as well as of the relational space where self and object meet.

There is considerable understanding of what occurs in the bipersonal interaction of patient and therapist in the psychoanalytic encounter, as well as a growing body of literature on countertransference (Bollas, 1987; Kernberg, 1979, 1984, 1987; Racker, 1968; Searles, 1975, 1979), along with more recent investigations of intersubjectivity (Atwood and Stolorow, 1984; Gill, 1982; Stolorow, Brandchaft, and Atwood, 1987). In the psychotherapeutic situation there is an area in which the boundaries of each participant are open to intersubjective relatedness. In conjoint therapy not only do the husband's and wife's boundaries open toward each other and the therapist, but the boundaries of the couple as a unit open toward the therapist.

I have illustrated the marital relational space in Figure 8.1, noting that this space is parallel to that which develops between the child and its primary caretaker. The space is the meeting of the self and other in marital therapy. It is within this relational space that the clues to what is experienced by the partners are discovered.

When the therapist observes the unfolding interaction and maintains a receptive capacity as to how he or she is used by each mate in the relational space between self and other, then various needs, affective states, and defenses emerge and become available for treatment. In order to operate therapeutically within that relational space, the therapist must be able to maintain a stance of open-minded curiosity about what is occurring within each of the participants in the therapeutic environment, listening for "news from within" and making some determination about its source. The internal experience of the therapist reflects the affective experience of the individual or the partners in the interactional space of the working relationship.

Empathy

Through observation of the interactional space, as well as a willingness to open boundaries to the couple, the therapist is able to assist in the transmutation of internal structures that affect relatedness. A major tool in this process is the therapist's ability to convey empathic understanding in a manner that can be taken in and used. Understanding alone will not be helpful to the couple or the individuals involved if it is thrust upon them in a way that is experienced as invasive. A theoretical interpretation based upon what has been learned by the therapist outside of the treatment situation is not likely to be experienced as an empathic response. Even if it is right, it must be conveyed in a way that can be incorporated instead of defended against.

Empathy does not take place in isolation and is not a unilateral intrapsychic phenomenon. It is an intersubjective phenomenon in which there is an inner experience of sharing and comprehending the momentary psychological state of the other (Schafer, 1959). Varying degrees of awareness may develop gradually over time or may emerge spontaneously as "an immediate flash" (Burke and Tansey, 1985, p. 372). Empathy is an aspect of a mutual transferential communicative process; it requires a freely oscillating pattern of identifications between the thoughts and feelings of the persons involved (Solomon, 1987).

The mental health field has long sought to understand this process more completely because of its importance to treatment. Fleiss (1942) referred to "trial identification" in which the therapist actively welcomes and openly receives transitory affective states in a manner similar to the way a theater audience eagerly awaits being stimulated and moved by the actors. Empathy, Fleiss wrote, is the ability to put oneself in the other's place, to step into his shoes, and to obtain in this way an inside knowledge that is almost firsthand. As the therapist opens up and willingly takes in on a "trial" basis whatever is sent by a patient, the process of understanding deepens. Boundaries are traversed through projective identification and the therapist's projective counter-identifications (Grotstein, 1981). In marital therapy this provides for a freely moving pattern of interactions between patient and therapist, between husband and wife, between couple and therapist.

"Empathy" is often used as a synonym for caring and sympathetic listening. Kohut (1984), however, has pointed out that empathy is not limited to a positive regard; in fact, an empathic understanding of another may be used to humiliate or destroy that person. Empathy is the ability to "read" the underlying affectivity of another and utilize the awareness of what the other is experiencing for benign or malevolent purposes. "In spite of any disagreement regarding the mechanism involved, the proponents of empathy through identification do us an important service by calling attention to the fact that there is an involuntary, unconsciously mediated transformation within . . . that is fundamental for the empathic experience" (Basch, 1983, p. 106).

"Identification" here takes place in an empathic encounter not with the other person *per se*, but with *what* he is experiencing (Basch, 1983). It is a matter of concluding that one's own affective state is either attuned to or replicates that of the other. This presumed similarity permits one to identify one's own affective position as representative of the other's mental state at a particular moment. In primary maternal preoccupation (Winnicott, 1971), mothers of newborns very accurately harmonize with the needs of their babies. In the developmental experience, "the parent transforms the infant's affective reactions into signals, consciously through reasoned evaluation of the significance of the child's facial expressions, cries, body posture, and movements, and, more importantly, unconsciously in reaction to the affective state that is produced in the parent by the child's affective expression" (Basch, 1983, p. 108). The reaction of the parent is based on inhibitions, conflicts in the area of affect receptivity, and the parent's own history of developmental arrests. This process of transmission of communications takes place also between patient and therapist, and in the unconscious communication that develops between intimate family partners.

Transference and Countertransference Between the Therapist and the Couple

Where the patient or couple is free to move in any direction—even in opposite directions at the same time—without the pull on the therapist being too strong, messages are communicated and information emerges from very deep levels. This is not as difficult as it might at first seem. At any point in treatment the dynamic interaction requires containment not of the totality of the patient's internal experiences, but only of the immediate relational spaces (see Figure 8.1).

How the therapist receives the patient's unwanted affectivity may become the basis for pathological collusions or a tool for empathic understanding. In marital therapy, the process of understanding the transference through empathic attunement helps the therapist to recognize and respond appropriately to unconscious needs and defend against unconscious anxiety. Questions such as, "At this moment, who is he to her?" "Who is she to him?" "Who am I to them?" "What function is each seeking from the other?" provide very important information about each of the mates and about the relationship. In the therapeutic setting it is possible answer these questions, to recognize the way couples deal within boundary issues, and to interact at the level where spouses are relating to each other. It is not necessary to respond to the totality of the relationship, only to that point of interaction between the two partners and between the meeting place of the relationship and the therapist's point of entry into the interaction.

It is in this sense of affect attunement with the unconscious aspects of another that the concept of countertransference is particularly useful. Like many terms in the psychoanalytic literature, countertransference has come to have several different meanings. I see countertransference as the therapist's totalistic reaction to the patient. Classical descriptions of the unconscious reactions of the therapist take them as something to be overcome through supervision or analysis. "Totalistic countertransference" (Kernberg, 1975), on the other hand, including all the conscious and unconscious reactions of the therapist to the patient, is a therapeutic instrument.

Figure 11.1 outlines countertransference issues based upon three factors: pathological and nonpathological transference reaction and various reality factors.

The classical model of countertransference includes the unconscious transference reactions the therapist brings to treatment, which are caused by unresolved issues in the therapist's life. This latter category of countertransference has been described in the psychoanalytic literature as composed of problems inherent in the therapist to be handled by case supervision or a return to analysis.

The patient's vulnerabilities, old injuries, projections, projective identifications, idealizations, expectations of the therapist, and narcissistic demand-

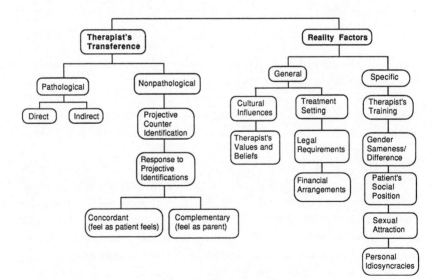

FIGURE 11.1
Totalistic Countertransference

ingness will invariably be reacted to by the therapist through "concordant" or "complementary" countertransference. Racker (1968) identified it as concordant countertransference when the therapist begins to experience what the patient is experiencing internally; for example, as a patient blandly describes severe abuse by her husband, the therapist's anger at the husband emerges. A therapist who becomes detached, sleepy, or bored may be responding concordantly to the patient's inner emotional deadness. When a patient has cut off and disavowed certain untenable internal experiences, the therapist may, through concordant countertransference, experience what the patient cannot feel. When the therapist's affect closely tracks the patient's affect, concordant identification becomes the basis of the therapist's empathy (Grayer and Sax, 1986).

Complementary countertransference occurs when the therapist has feelings that relate to the patient's parent or other early figures. Racker (1968) suggested that complementary countertransference is produced by the patient's treating the therapist as an internal (projected) object. The therapist in this case feels treated as, rather than identified with, the patient's internal object representations (Grayer and Sax, 1986). The therapist comes to identify him/herself as this object, for example, a parent or mate who is the counterpart to the patient's feelings. The therapist may momentarily feel like, and begin to behave as, the parent. While we recognize that it is acting-out if the therapist becomes angry, withholding, or seductive in a countertransferential reaction to the patient's provocative behavior, we are less aware of the countertransference that occurs in response to patients' idealizations, wishes for affirmation, or attempts to model themselves after their therapists.

Reality issues of therapists' and patients' lives, including social and cultural issues influencing their values and beliefs, cannot be ignored. Included here are also issues of the treatment setting, especially financial arrangements and legal requirements. Additional reality factors related to countertransference include the therapist's training and experience, gender, the financial and social positions of patient and therapist, sexual attraction, and the personal idiosyncracies of patient and therapist.

Countertransference as a Tool of Treatment

Since countertransference can be used as a communicative tool to obtain important information about the inner emotional constellation of the patient, therapists need to examine their own countertransference openly and honestly and, where it will help, communicate certain aspects of their countertransference feelings to patients (Searles, 1979; Skynner, 1981).

"There are times when the therapist may feel himself to be possessed, indeed, even overwhelmed or threatened with the loss of his identity and sanity, and may carry around such disturbing projections within himself for quite long periods before they suddenly disappear and return to the patient" (Skynner, 1976, p. 79). In this process, the therapist may internalize the patient's problem for a time, work on it, and hand it back detoxified so that the patient can reincorporate it safely.

I recall one couple who vividly illustrate the emotional dangers attendant to the therapist's role. The husband was chairman of a conglomerate corporation, a super-successful jet-setter. His wife, a 32-year-old South American from a political family, fundamentally bright and capable, was extremely fragmented and had been hearing voices. Her symptoms frightened her and she wanted to go home to South America.

I had a strange experience of confusion around them, of momentarily forgetting names and losing track of facts. I usually trust my internal reactions and often respond intuitively without checking my every word. Why, then, did I have these insecurities with them, as though I were going to make some major error that would disrupt treatment? Why did I continue to expect that something was going to go wrong? How much was related to my own wish to be seen as highly competent and accepted by these interesting people? To what extent was I reacting to their unstated anxieties and needs below the façade of success? I wondered.

I told them that I was having some doubts about my ability to help them and thought we might spend some time discussing this, as I certainly did not want to waste their time and money. The wife began by reassuring me. As we talked further, she spoke of her fear that I would give up on them because they were so impossible, and then they would be "thrown away" and left with no help. As she related these feelings to her earlier terror of being abandoned, the husband said that he had been wondering the same thing that I was, whether or not I would really be able to understand. "I am a very complicated man," he said, "I send out smoke signals to make sure I keep others off balance. I think I can do it to you also. So you probably cannot help me." As he spoke there seemed to be a combination of pride and sadness. Can no one take care of his need then? I wondered. Does he stay safe by always being alone? What is so dangerous that he always must maintain power over others? How does it affect his marriage?

From there our work began. The result was a treatment which lasted over three years and ended with their marriage strengthened, and with the couple deciding to return to South America. I was struck by the fluctuations in my own feelings during the time we worked together. As we went through intense, oscillating experiences—first the husband, then the wife, then the relationship—at varying points in the therapy, I became aware of how I shifted between confusion, anger, admiration, and affection. Although my shifting emotions were not generally verbally identified as such to the couple, they had a considerable effect on my responses. Whether my feeling of great fondness for them at the point of termination was the result of the successful outcome, or whether the success in treatment was based upon their awareness that their well-being was truly important to me, is open to speculation. I was aware of a mixture of pleasure and loss as we parted for the last time.

Countertransference With Narcissistic Disorders

One of the main dangers in dealing with narcissistic patients is that they will engage in behaviors that make therapists feel discounted and angry while at the same time demanding total involvement and confirming responses. No matter how hard a therapist tries, the transference process invariably engenders countertransference reactions—love or hate or some mixture of intense feelings that could adversely affect conjoint therapy. A very important countertransference factor that invariably affects the therapeutic relationship is the therapist's own emotional set. The personal history of the therapist, the therapist's own therapy, affects his or her expectations of self and others and becomes a role model for treatment.

Occasionally, a husband and wife combine to attack and confuse the therapist. "This therapy isn't working. We don't think you can help us. We've been coming for six months and it's a waste of time. We're thinking of going someplace else." It is natural for a therapist in such a situation to feel useless or worse—after all, one's professional competency has been challenged. The feelings can lead a well-intentioned professional to find a way to terminate with a couple or an individual too soon. It is necessary to explore with the mates their sense of hopelessness and disappointment. If they leave they will still experience a combination of relief and loss.

A chronic danger in treating both narcissistic individuals and couples is the fatigue produced by the heavy demands upon the therapist. A tired therapist retaliates by losing interest and tuning out. Therapists can become distracted and feel overloaded, not only because of the material being presented but also because of anxiety that they will be overburdened or overwhelmed by the patient's needs. The unconscious wish of some narcissistic patients is that spouse and therapist give up their own identity and exist only for the patient.

As has been noted, many factors can cause a therapist to align with one spouse at the expense of the other, to the detriment of the treatment. One partner's façade of grandiosity or narcissistic demands may drive the therapist into alignment with the other. This can increase the level of the first partner's rage, even to the point of dropping out of treatment. Even if the unfavored spouse stays in the treatment for a time, there is a defensive against narcissistic injury caused by the sessions. Feelings of shame or humiliation may emerge as one feels blame and the other feels guilt. The blamed partner may be labeled "resistant" or may be identified as the "disturbed" one.

THE MARRIAGE AS PATIENT

The therapist need not be committed to seeing that the couple stay together no matter what happens, but a therapeutic stance as spokesman for the marriage permits somebody to speak for the relationship without putting that burden on one partner or the other. When one of the partners clearly wants out, the therapist can help the partners deal with the implications of separation and divorce. However, to say that it does not matter whether a marriage works out or not when a couple has come for marital therapy seems similar to saying that is does not matter whether or not a patient in individual treatment improves.

When a therapist accepts a case for marital therapy, the therapist has an obligation not to select which mate is "right" and which is "wrong" in their mutual difficulties. The issue should not be refocused on whether individual growth may be promoted by terminating the relationship, although referral to individual psychotherapy may provide a suitable arena for such questions. Individual growth may be a valid subject, but when the marital therapist chooses such a refocusing of the treatment issue, it can easily lead to a conflict of goals. Very often therapy evolves into resolving a basic conflict between what is good for the marriage and what is best for one or both of the individuals.

Many adults today are reconsidering whether or not the rewards of marriage compensate for the efforts involved. Some decide not to invest their emotional energies in marriage. They choose alternate ways to meet their needs for emotional connections and loving relationships. But those who have chosen to marry and wish to remain married may seek out therapy when relationship problems become more than they can handle. When couples seek therapy for the marriage, the *marriage* is the patient and the therapist's commitment is to work toward its healing. The role of the marital therapist is as an advocate for the marriage primarily, and for individual growth and development within the security of an ongoing relationship. It has been a basic assumption of this book that solid marital relationships are of such value that we need to develop a theory of dynamic marital therapy as a specific discipline with a focus on realizing the potential of a secure, intimate relationship for emotional health. Deepening the bonds of intimacy will beneficially affect the lives of the partners, the family, and society.

References

Andreas-Salome, L. (1962). The dual orientation of narcissism. *Psychoanalytic Quarterly, 31*, 1–30.

Atwood, G. E., & Stolorow, R. D. (1984). *Structures of subjectivity: Explorations in psychoanalytic phenomenology*. Hillsdale, New Jersey: The Analytic Press.

Basch, M. (1983). Empathic understanding: A review of the concept and some theoretical considerations. *Journal of the American Psychoanalytic Association, 31*, 101–125.

Basch, M. (1985). Interpretation: Toward a developmental model. In A. Goldberg (Ed.), *Progress in self psychology: Vol. 1* (pp. 33–42). New York: Guilford Press.

Beck, R. L. (1987). Redirecting blaming in marital therapy. *Clinical Social Work Journal, 15*(2), 148–158.

Bergmann, M. S. (1987). *The anatomy of loving*. New York: Columbia University Press.

Bernard, J. (1972). *The future of marriage*. New Haven, CT: Yale University Press.

Bion, W. R. (1961). *Experiences in groups*. London: Tavistock.

Bion, W. R. (1967). *Second thoughts: Selected papers on psychoanalysis*. New York: Jason Aronson.

Bion, W. R. (1977). *Seven servants*. New York: Jason Aronson.

Blumstein, P., & Schwartz, P. (1983). *American couples*. New York: William Morrow.

Bollas, C. (1983). Expressive use of the countertransference. *Contemporary Psychoanalysis, 19*(1), 1–34.

Bollas, C. (1985, October). *A loving hatred*. Presentation at the Newport Institute for Psychoanalytic Studies.

Bollas, C. (1987). *The shadow of the object: Psychoanalysis of the unthought known*. New York: Columbia University Press.

Boszormenyi-Nagy, I., & Krasner, B. (1986). *Between give and take: A clinical guide to contextual therapy*. New York: Brunner/Mazel.

Boszormenyi-Nagy, I., & Spark, G. M. (1984). *Invisible loyalties: Reciprocity in intergenerational family therapy*. New York: Brunner/Mazel.

Bowen, M. (1966). The use of family theory in clinical practice. *Comparative Psychiatry, 7*, 345–374.

Bowen, M. (1972). On the differentiation of self. In J. Framo (Ed.), *Family interaction:*

Dialogue between family researchers and family therapists (pp. 11–173). New York: Springer.

Bowen, M. (1976). Theory in the practice of psychotherapy. In P. J. Guerin (Ed.), *Family therapy: Theory and practice* (pp. 42–91). New York: Garner Press.

Bowen, M. (1978). *Family therapy in clinical practice*. New York: Jason Aronson.

Bowlby, J. (1969). *Attachment and loss* (Vols. 1–2). New York: Basic Books.

Brandchaft, B. (1983). The negativism of the negative therapeutic reaction and the psychology of the self. In A. Goldberg (Ed.), *The Future of psychoanalysis* (pp. 327–359). New York: International Universities Press.

Brazelton, T. B. (1969). *Infants and mothers—differences in development*. New York: Dell Publishing.

Brenner, C. (1974). On the nature and development of affects: A unified theory. *Psychoanalytic Quarterly, 43*, 532–556.

Brenner, C. (1975). Affects and psychic conflict. *Psychoanalytic Quarterly, 44*, 5–28.

Brown, S. (1984). *Countertransference in treatment of couples*. Paper presented at University of California conference "Psychodynamic marital therapy," Los Angeles, CA.

Burke, W. F., & Tansey, M. J. (1985). Projective identification and countertransference turmoil: Disruptions in the empathic process. *Contemporary Psychoanalysis, 21*, 372–401.

Burlingham, D. (1967). Empathy between infant and mother. *Journal of the American Psychoanalytic Association, 16*, 675–696.

Cancian, F. (1987). *Love in America: Gender and self-development*. Cambridge: Cambridge University Press.

Cassiver, E. (1955). *The philosophy of symbolic forms of language* (Vol. 1). New Haven, CT: Yale University Press.

Chasseguet-Smirgel, J. (1984). *Creativity and perversion*. New York: W. W. Norton.

Clynes, M. (1980). The communication of emotion: Theory of sentics. In R. Plutchik and H. Kellerman (Eds.), *Emotion: Theory, research, and experience* (pp. 271–301). New York: Academic Press.

Cooper, A. M. (1986). What men fear: The facade of castration anxiety. In G. I. Fogel, F. M. Lane, & R. S. Liebert (Eds.), *The psychology of men: New psychoanalytic perspectives* (pp. 113–130). New York: Basic Books.

Deutsch, H. (1970). Occult processes occurring during psychoanalysis. In G. Devereux (Ed.), *Psychoanalysis and the occult* (pp. 133–146). New York: International University Press. (Original work published in 1926)

Dicks, H. V. (1953). Experience with marital tensions in the psychological clinic. *British Journal of Medicine, 26*, 181.

Dicks, H. V. (1967). *Marital tension: Clinical studies toward a psychological theory of interaction*. London: Routledge and Kegan Paul.

Emde, R. N. (1980). Toward a psychoanalytic theory of affect. In S. I. Greenspan and G. H. Pollock (Eds.), *Infancy and early childhood. The course of life: Psychoanalytic contributions towards understanding personality development* (Vol. 1, pp. 63–112). Washington, D. C.: National Institute of Mental Health.

Epstein, S. (1973). The self-concept revisited. *American Psychologist, 28*, 404.

Escalona, S. (1968). *The roots of individuality*. Chicago: Aldine.

Fairbairn, W. R. (1952). *Psychosomatic studies of the personality*. London: Tavistock.

Fairbairn, W. R. (1954). Schizoid factors in the personality. In *An object relations theory of personality* (pp. 3–27). New York: Basic Books. (Original work published 1940).

Fairbairn, W. R. (1954). *An object relations theory of personality*. New York: Basic Books.

Fleiss, R. (1942). The metapsychology of the analyst. *Psychoanalytic Quarterly, 11*, 211–227.

Framo, J. L. (1980). The integration of marital therapy with sessions with family of origin. In A. S. Gurman & D. P. Kniskern (Eds.), *Handbook of family therapy* (pp. 133–158). New York: Brunner/Mazel.

Framo, J. L. (1982). *Explorations in marital and family therapy*. New York: Springer.

Freud, S. (1953). The interpretations of dreams. In J. Strachey (Ed. and Trans.), *The standard edition of the complete psychological works of Sigmund Freud* (Vols. 4–5). New York: W. W. Norton. (Original work published in 1900)

Freud, S. (1955). Group psychology and the analysis of the ego. In J. Strachey (Ed. and Trans.), *The standard edition of the complete psychological works of Sigmund Freud* (Vol. 18 pp. 67–143). New York: W. W. Norton. (Original work published 1921)

Freud, S. (1958). Formulations on the two principles of mental functioning. In J. Strachey (Ed. and Trans.), *The standard edition of the complete psychological works of Sigmund Freud* (Vol. 12 pp. 213–226). New York: W. W. Norton. (Original work published 1911)

Gaylin, W. (1984). *The rage within: Anger in modern life*. New York: Simon and Schuster.

Gill, M. (1982). *Analysis of transference: Theory and technique, Vol. 1*. New York: International Universities Press.

Gilligan, C. (1982). *In a different voice*. Cambridge, Mass: Harvard University Press.

Giovacchini, P. (1987). The "unreasonable" patient and the psychotic transference in the borderline patient. In J. Grotstein, M. Solomon, & J. Lang (Eds.), *The borderline patient: Emerging concepts in diagnosis, etiology, psychodynamics, and treatment* (pp. 59–68). New Jersey: The Analytic Press.

Giovacchini, P. (1965). Treatment of marital disharmonies: The classical approach. In B. Green (Ed.), *The psychotherapies of marital disharmony*. NY: Free Press.

Goldklank, S. (1986). My family made me do it: The influence of family therapists' family of origin on their occupational choice. *Family Process, 25*, 309–324.

Grayer, E., & Sax, P. (1986). A model for the diagnostic and therapeutic use of countertransference. *Clinical Social Work, 14*(4), 295–309.

Green, A. (1977). Conceptions of affect. *International Journal of Psychoanalysis, 58*, 129–156.

Greenberg, J. R., & Mitchell, S. (1983). *Object relations in psychoanalytic theory*. Cambridge: Harvard University Press.

Grotstein, J. (1981). *Splitting and projective identification*. New York: Jason Aronson.

Grotstein, J. (1987). The borderline as a disorder of self-regulation. In J. Grotstein, M. Solomon, & J. Lang (Eds.), *The borderline patient: Emerging concepts in diagnosis, etiology, psychodynamics, and treatment* (pp. 347–385). Hillsdale, NJ: The Analytic Press.

Grotstein, J., Solomon, M., & Lang, J. (1987). *The borderline patient: Emerging concepts in diagnosis, etiology, psychodynamics, and treatment*. Hillsdale, NJ: The Analytic Press.

Grunberger, B. (1979). *Narcissism: Psychoanalytic essays* (J. S. Diamanti, Trans.). New York: International Universities Press.

Guidubaldi, J., & Perry, J. D. (1985). Divorce and mental health sequelae for children: A two year follow-up of a nationwide sample. *Journal of the American Academy of Child Psychiatry, 24*, 531–537.

Gurman, A. S. (1978). Contemporary marital therapy: A critique and comparative analysis of psychoanalytic, behavioral and systems theory approaches. In T. J. Paolino & B. S. McCrady (Eds.), *Marriage and marital therapy* (pp. 445–566). New York: Brunner/Mazel.

Gurman, A. S. (1977). The patient's perception of the therapeutic relationship. In A. Gurman & A. Ragin (Eds.), *Effective psychotherapy: A handbook of research* (pp. 00–00). New York: Pergamon Press.

Gurman, A. S. (1979). Dimensions of marital therapy: A comparative analysis. *Journal of Marital and Family Therapy, 5*, 5–16.

Gurman, A. S. (1980). Behavioral marriage therapy in the 1980's: The challenge of integration. *American Journal of Family Therapy, 8*, 86–96.

Guttman, H. A. (1987). Transference and countertransference in marital therapy. In L. F. Frelick & E. M. Waring (Eds.), *Marital therapy in psychiatric practice: An overview* (pp. 136–164). New York: Brunner/Mazel.

Hall, E. T. (1966). *The hidden dimension*. Garden City, N.Y.: Macmillan.

Harrison, E. (1985). *Masks of the universe*. New York: Macmillan.

Hetherington, E. M., Cox, M. & Cox, R. (1985). Long term effects of divorce and remarriage on the adjustment of children. *Journal of the American Academy of Child Psychiatry, 24*, 518–530.

Hetherington, E. M., & Parke, R. D. (1979). *Child Psychology: A contemporary viewpoint*. New York: McGraw-Hill.

Hildebrandt, H. (1986–87). *The newly promoted executive*. Ann Arbor: University of Michigan, School of Business, Division of Research.

Hildebrandt, H. (1987). *A review of managers in U.S. industries*. Ann Arbor: University of Michigan, School of Business, Division of Research.

Hite, S. (1987). *The Hite report, women and love: A cultural revolution in progress*. New York: Knopf.

Horner, A. (1986). *Being and loving*. New York: Jason Aronson.

Jackson, D., & Lederer, W. (1968). *Mirages of marriage*. New York: W. W. Norton.

Johnson, S. M. (1987). *Humanizing the narcissistic style*. New York: W. W. Norton.

Joseph, B. (1987). Projective identification: Clinical aspects. In J. Sandler (Ed.), *Projection, interjection, projective identification* (pp. 65–76). Madison, Conn: International Universities Press.

Kernberg, O. (1979). *Object relations theory and clinical psychoanalysis*. New York: Jason Aronson.

Kernberg, O. F. (1984). *Severe personality disorders: Psychotherapeutic strategies*. New Haven: Yale University Press.

Kernberg, O. F. (1975). *Borderline conditions and pathological narcissism*. New York: Jason Aronson.

Kernberg, O. (1987). Projection and projective identification: Developmental and clinical aspects. *Journal of the American Psychoanalytic Association, 35*, 795–820.

Kernberg, P. (1984). *The psychological assessment of children with borderline personality organization*. Paper presented to the American Psychoanalytic Association, NY.

Kerr, M., & Bowen, M. (1988). *Family evaluation: An approach based on Bowen Theory*. New York: W. W. Norton.

Klein, M. (1946). Notes on some schizoid mechanisms. *International Journal of Psychoanalysis, 33*, 433–438.

Klein, M. (1975). *Envy and gratitude*. New York: Delacorte Press.

Klein, S. (1981). Autistic phenomena in neurotic patients. In J. Grotstein (Ed.), *Do I dare disturb the universe?* (pp. 103–114). Beverly Hills, CA: Caesura Press.

Kohut, H. (1971). *Analysis of the self*. New York: International Universities Press.

Kohut, H. (1977). *Restoration of the self*. New York: International Universities Press.

Kohut, H. (1984). *How does analysis cure?* Edited by A. Goldberg with P. E. Stepansky. Chicago: University of Chicago Press.

Kubie, L. (1956). Psychoanalysis and marriage: Practical and theoretical issues. In V. Eisenstein (Ed.), *Neurotic interaction in marriage* (pp. 10–43). New York: Basic Books.

Lang, J. (1985). *Passionate attachments*. Lecture given at Lectures on Passionate Attachments Continuing Education Seminars. Los Angeles, California.

Langs, R. (1976a). *The bipersonal field*. New York: Jason Aronson.

Langs, R. (1976b). *The therapeutic interaction: Vol. 2*. New York: Jason Aronson.

Langs, R. (1983). *Unconscious communication in everyday life*. New York: Jason Aronson.

Lansky, M. (1980). On blame. *International Journal of Psychoanalytic Psychotherapy, 8*, 429–456.

Lansky, M. (1981). Treatment of the narcissistically vulnerable marriage. In M. Lansky (Ed.), *Family therapy and major psychopathology* (pp. 163–182). New York: Grune & Stratton.

Lansky, M. (1985). *Preoccupation and pathogenic distance regulation.* Paper presented at University of California conference, "Psychodynamic marital therapy," Los Angeles, CA.

Lansky, M. (1987). Shame and the families of borderline patients. In J. Grotstein, M. Solomon, & J. Lang (Eds.), *The borderline patient: Emerging concepts in diagnosis, etiology, psychodynamics and treatment* (Vol. 2, pp. 187–200). New Jersey: The Analytic Press.

Lasch, C. (1979). *The culture of narcissism: American life in an age of diminishing expectations.* New York: Norton.

Lachkar, J. (1985). Narcissistic/borderline couples: Theoretical implications for treatment. *Dynamic Psychotherapy, 3*(2), 109–125.

Levinson, D. L. (1978). *The seasons of a man's life.* New York: Knopf.

Lichtenberg, J. D. (1983). *Psychoanalysis and infant research.* Hillsdale, New Jersey: Analytic Press.

Mahler, M. S., Pine, F., & Bergman, A. (1975). *The psychological birth of the human infant: Symbiosis and individuation.* New York: Basic Books.

Masterson, J. F. (1981). *The narcissistic and borderline disorders: An integrative approach.* New York: Brunner/Mazel.

McDermott, J. F. (1970). Divorce and its psychiatric sequelae in children. *Archives of General Psychiatry, 23*, 421–428.

McDougall, J. (1986). *Theaters of the mind: Illusion of truth on the psychoanalytic stage.* New York: Basic Books.

McDougall, J. (in press). *Theaters of the body.* New York: W. W. Norton.

McGoldrick, M., & Gerson, R. (1985). *Genograms in family assessment.* New York: W. W. Norton.

Miller, A. (1981). *Prisoners of childhood.* New York: Basic Books.

Nadelson, C. C., & Paolino, T. J. (1978). Marital therapy from a psychoanalytic perspective. In T. J. Paolini & B. S. McCrady (Eds.), *Marriage and marital therapy: Psychoanalytic, behavioral and systems perspectives* (pp. 89–165). New York: Brunner/Mazel.

Napier, A. Y. (1978). The rejection-intrusion pattern: A central family dynamic. *Journal of Marriage and Family Counseling, 4*, 5–12.

Nass, G., Libby, R. W., & Fisher, M. (1981). *Sexual choices: An introduction to human sexuality.* Monterey, CA.: Wadsworth Health Sciences Division.

Nathanson, D. L. (1987). *The many faces of shame.* New York: Guilford Press.

Ogden, T. H. (1982). *Projective identification and psychoanalytic technique.* New York: Jason Aronson.

Ornstein, A., & Ornstein, P. (1985). Parenting as a function of the adult self: A psychoanalytic developmental perspective. In J. Anthony & G. H. Pollock (Eds.), *Parental influences in health and disease* (pp. 183–234). Boston: Little Brown and Company.

Palombo, J. (1987). Self object transferences in the treatment of borderline neurocognitively impaired children. In J. Grotstein, M. Solomon, & J. Lang (Eds.), *The borderline patient: Emerging concepts in diagnosis, etiology. psychodynamics and treatment* (Vol. 1, pp. 317–346). New Jersey: The Analytic Press.

Perls, F. (1969). *Gestalt therapy verbatim.* Moab, Utah: Real People Press.

Person, E. S. (1988). *Dreams of love and fateful encounters.* New York: W. W. Norton.

Pine, F. (1986a). "The symbiotic phase" in light of current research. *Bulletin of the Menninger Clinic, 50*, 564–569.

Pine, Fred, (1986b). On the development of the "borderline child to be". *American Journal of Orthopsychiatry, 56*(3), 450–457.

Racker, H. (1968). The meaning and uses of countertransference. In H. Racker (Ed.), *Transference and countertransference.* London: Hogarth Press. (Original work published in 1957)

Rapaport, D. (1967). On the psychoanalytic theory of affects. In M. Gill (Ed.), *Collected papers* (pp. 476–512). New York: Basic Books. (Original work published in 1953)

Rinsley, D. B. (1982). *Borderline and other self disorders: A developmental and object relations perspective*. New York: Jason Aronson.

Sacks, O. (1985). *The man who mistook his wife for a hat*. New York: Summit Books.

Sacksteder, J. L., Schwartz, D. P., & Akabane, Y. (1987). *Attachment and the therapeutic process: Essays in honor of Otto Allen Will, Jr.* Madison, Connecticut: International Universities Press.

Sager, C. J., Gundlach, R., & Kremer, M. (1968). The married in treatment. *Archives of General Psychiatry, 19*, 205–217.

Sandler, J., (1987). *Projection, interjection, projective identification*. Madison, Connecticut: International Universities Press.

Schafer, R. (1959). Generative empathy in the treatment situation. *Psychoanalytic Quarterly, 28*, 347–373.

Scharf, M. (1987). *Intimate partners*. New York: Random House.

Scharff, D., & Scharff, J. (1987). *Object relations family therapy*. New Jersey: Jason Aronson.

Searles, H. (1975). The patient as therapist to his analyst. In P. Giovacchini (Ed.), *Tactics and techniques of psychoanalytic therapy* (Vol. 2, pp. 95–151). New York: Jason Aronson.

Searles, H. (1979). *Countertransference and related subjects*. New York: International University Press.

Shor, J., & Sanville, J. (1978). *Illusion in loving*. Los Angeles: Double Helix Press.

Skynner, A. C. R. (1976). *Systems of family and marital psychotherapy*. New York: Brunner/Mazel.

Skynner, A. C. R. (1981). An open systems group analytic approach to family therapy. In A. S. Gurman & D. P. Kniskern (Eds.), *Handbook of family therapy* (pp. 39–85). New York: Brunner/Mazel.

Slipp, S. (1984). *Object relations: A dynamic bridge between individual and family treatment*. new York: Jason Aronson.

Solomon, M. (1985). Treatment of narcissistic and borderline disorders in marital therapy: Suggestions toward an enhanced therapeutic approach. *Clinical Social Work, July, 1985, 141–156*.

Solomon, M. (1987). Application of psychoanalytic treatments for the nonanalytic practitioner. In J. Grotstein, M. Solomon, & J. Lang, (Eds.), *The Borderline Patient*. New Jersey: Analytic Press.

Solomon, M. (1988a). Self psychology and marital therapy. *International Journal of Family Psychiatry*.

Solomon, M. (1988b). Treatment of narcissistic vulnerability in marital therapy, (Ed) in Goldberg, *Progress in Self Psychology*, Volume IV, New Jersey: Analytic Press.

Spitz, R. (1965). *The first year of life*. New York: International Universities Press.

Stern, D. (1985). *The interpersonal world of the infant*. New York: Basic Books.

Stolorow, R. D., & Lachmann, F. M. (1980). *Psychoanalysis of developmental arrests: Theory and treatment*. New York: International Universities Press.

Stolorow, R. D., Brandchaft, B., & Atwood, G. E. (1987). *Psychoanalytic treatment: An intersubjective approach*. Hillsdale, New Jersey: The Analytic Press.

Stone, M. (1980). *The borderline syndromes*. New York: McGraw-Hill.

Sullivan, H. S. (1953). *The interpersonal world of psychiatry*. New York: W. W. Norton.

Tansey, M. H., & Burke, W. F. (1985). Projective identification and the empathic process: Interactional communications. *Contemporary Psychoanalysis, 21*, 42–67.

Tolpin, M. (1983). Corrective emotional experience: A self psychological reevaluation. In A. Goldberg (Ed.), *The future of psychoanalysis: Essays in honor of Heinz Kohut* (pp. 363–379). New York: International Universities Press.

Tomkins, S. S. (1980). Affect as amplification: Some modifications in theory. In R. Plutchik & H. Kellerman (Eds.), *Emotion: Theory, research, and experience* (pp. 141–164). New York: Academic Press.

Tomkins, S. S. (1987). Shame. In D. L. Nathanson (Ed.), *The many faces of shame* (pp. 133–161). New York: Guilford Press.

Tustin, F. (1987). *Autistic barriers in neurotic patients*. New Haven, CT: Yale University Press.

Wachtel, E. F., & Wachtel, P. L. (1986). *Family dynamics in individual psychotherapy*. New York: Guilford Press.

Wallerstein, J. S. (1985). Children of divorce: Preliminary report of a ten-year follow-up of older children and adolescents. *Journal of the American Academy of Child Psychiatry, 24,* 545–553.

Watzlawick, P., Beavin, J. H., & Jackson, D. D. (1967). *Pragmatics of human communication*. New York: W. W. Norton.

Will, O. A. (1980). Schizophrenia: Psychological treatment. In H. Kaplan, A. M. Fredman, & B. J. Sadock (Eds.), *Comprehensive textbook of psychiatry III* (Vol 2, pp. 1217–1240). Baltimore, MD: Williams and Wilkins.

Will, O. A. (1987). Illuminations of the human condition. In J. L. Sacksteder, D. S. Schwartz, & Y. Akabane (Eds.), *Attachment and the therapeutic process: Essays in honor of Otto Allen Will, Jr.* (pp. 241–261). Madison, Connecticut: International Universities Press.

Willi, J. (1982). *Couples in collusion*. NY, London: Jason Aronson.

Willi, J. (1984). *Dynamics of couples therapy*. NY, London: Jason Aronson.

Winnicott, D. W. (1958). Pediatrics and childhood neurosis. In D. Winnicott (Ed.), *Collected papers: Through pediatrics to psychoanalysis* (pp. 316–321). London: Tavistock Publications. (Original work published 1956)

Winnicott, D. W. (1965). *The maturational process and the facilitating environment: Studies in the theory of emotional development*. New York: International Universities Press.

Winnicott, D. W. (1971). *Playing and reality*. Middlesex, England: Penguin.

Winnicott, D. W. (1986). *Home is where we start from*. New York: W. W. Norton.

Wynne, L., Ryckoff, I., Day, J., & Hirsch, S. (1958). Pseudo-mutuality in the family relations of schizophrenics. *Psychiatry, 21,* 205–220.

Wynne, L. (1987). Mutuality and pseudomutuality reconsidered: Implications for therapy and a theory of development of relational systems. In J. L. Sacksteder, D. S. Schwartz, & Y. Akabane (Eds.), *Attachment and the therapeutic process: Essays in honor of Otto Allen Will, Jr.* (pp. 81–98). Madison, Connecticut: International Universities Press.

Zill, N. (1983). *Happy, healthy and insecure*. New York: Doubleday.

Index